ELECTRONIC HEALTH RECORDS

Strategies for Implementation

Margret Amatayakul, MBA, RHIA, CHPS, FHIMSS

Michael R. Cohen, MM, FHIMSS

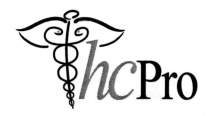

Electronic Health Records: Strategies for Implementation is published by HCPro, Inc.

Copyright 2004 HCPro, Inc.

All rights reserved. Printed in the United States of America   5   4   3   2   1

ISBN 1-57839-517-8

Margret Amatayakul, MBA, RHIA, CHPS, FHIMSS, Author
Michael R. Cohen, MM, FHIMSS, Co-author
Ilene G. MacDonald, Senior Managing Editor
Jean St. Pierre, Creative Director
Mike Mirabello, Senior Graphic Artist
Crystal Beland, Layout Artist
Mike Michaud, Layout Artist
Laura Godinho, Cover Designer
Lauren McLeod, Group Publisher
Suzanne Perney, Publisher

Advice given is general. Readers should consult professional counsel for specific legal, ethical, or clinical questions.

Arrangements can be made for quantity discounts. For more information, contact:

HCPro, Inc.
P.O. Box 1168
Marblehead, MA 01945
Telephone: 800/650-6787 or 781-639-1872
Fax: 781/639-2982
E-mail: *customerservice@hcpro.com*

Visit HCPro, Inc., at our Web sites: *www.hcmarketplace.com* and *www.hcpro.com*

12/2004
20194

Contents

About the Authors

Margret Amatayakul, MBA, RHIA, CHPS, FHIMSS

Margret Amatayakul, MBA, RHIA, CHPS, FHIMSS, is president of Margret\A Consulting, LLC, a firm dedicated to providing effective and efficient solutions to today's information management and systems issues. Her MBA from the University of Illinois at Chicago concentrated on marketing and finance. She has also taken coursework from the Illinois Institute of Technology in systems analysis.

Margret "A" helped found and was the executive director of the Computer-based Patient Record Institute (CPRI), which was a recommendation in the Institute of Medicine (IOM) patient record study (April 1991). CPRI is now part of the Healthcare Information Management and Systems Society (HIMSS), continuing the Davies Recognition Program for exemplary implementations of EHRs that was initiated during Margret's tenure.

Margret has a long and extensive career history of working in the field of EHRs and associated standards, including ASTM and HL7. She serves on the HIMSS Board of Directors and its Privacy and Security Steering Committee. She has been a contractor to the National Committee on Vital and Health Statistics (NCVHS), assisting them in developing their recommendations on uniform data standards for patient medical record information and electronic prescribing.

As the associate executive director of the American Health Information Management Association (AHIMA), Margret was responsible for overseeing academic preparation, continuing education, and certification, as well as the association's early advocacy efforts. Margret has also been an associate professor at the University of Illinois at Chicago and director of health information management at the Illinois Eye and Ear Infirmary. She is currently an adjunct faculty member in the health informatics masters program at the College of St. Scholastica, and on the advisory committee to its Title III grant, which, in partnership with a major EHR vendor, focuses on integrating computer-based clinical information system applications into health sciences professional curricula.

Michael R. Cohen, MM, FHIMSS

Michael R. Cohen, MM, FHIMSS, has more than 25 years of experience in healthcare information systems and has established a reputation as one of the leading authorities on the healthcare IT marketplace.

Mike has experience as a consultant, information systems vendor, and hospital administrator. He was Vice President at Sheldon I. Dorenfest & Associates, a Senior Manager at Arthur Young & Company (now Cap Gemini Ernst and Young), a marketing support specialist at McDonnell Douglas Automation Company (now McKesson/HBOC), a manager at Arthur Andersen and Co. (now Accenture), and an administrator at Cook County Hospital in Chicago.

He is active in the Healthcare Information Management Systems Society (HIMSS) and is a member of the Healthcare Financial Management Association (HFMA), American College of Healthcare Executives (ACHE), and National Association of Healthcare Consultants (NAHC). He is a frequent speaker and author of a variety of information systems topics, is a past chairman of the First Illinois HFM Chapter's Information Systems Committee, and serves on the editorial board of "ADVANCE for Health Information Executives." Mike received his Masters in Management (equivalent to an MBA/MHA) degree with concentrations in Health Care Administration and Finance from the Northwestern Graduate School of Management.

Acknowledgements

Special thanks to the following individuals for contributing their thoughts and time to this project:

John Schreier, Elgin, IL, contributed to the development of Chapter 4. He is an independent consultant with more than 20 years experience as a director of information systems in healthcare organizations. He focuses on planning and implementing electronic patient record systems, including computerized physician order entry.

Lawrence Pawola, PharmD, MBA, contributed to Chapter 5. He is an associate professor of health informatics and pharmacy practice, School of Biomedical and Health Information Sciences, College of Applied Health Sciences, University of Illinois at Chicago, and president of Lincolnshire Consulting Associates, LLC.

Introduction

Why a book on EHR implementation?

There are numerous articles and other reference materials on electronic health records (EHR): what they are, how to select them, why they are important, and what standards are needed for them. There are also other general reference works on information system design. And then, of course, there are implementation guides and installation instructions from the EHR vendor. But there is very little overall guidance on implementation of EHR systems that touches on the people, policy, and process of actually putting in place an EHR system.

EHR systems have inherent qualities that make their implementation unique. In addition, many people who become involved in EHR implementation typically have never been involved in any other information system implementation or have not put in place systems that touch the core business of health care as do EHRs.

Who should read this book?

In general, there are three categories of individuals in health care who would benefit specifically:

- Information systems project managers who have helped healthcare organizations carry out financial, administrative, and departmental operations systems, such as laboratory information systems, document imaging systems, or rehabilitation service systems. This book will help you understand the scope and complexity of both an information system that focuses on the core business of health care and persons who have generally not used an information system in the past.

- Healthcare organization clinical and ancillary staff who find themselves for the first time on an EHR steering committee, project team, or in some other way involved with the implementation of an EHR. You may be your department's designated "super user." This book should help you understand the planning, infrastructure preparedness, workflow redesign and process changes, and system build activities with which you will need to be involved.

- Information systems analysts who have a solid background in computers and systems outside of health care, and who have been tapped to assist a healthcare organization implement its EHR. This may be small community hospital, clinic, or other specialty facility that does not have extensive information system resources or a large information system department. This book should help you focus on the special issues facing health care as you implement your EHR system.

How can this book help with EHR implementation?

Although the concept of EHR has been around for many years in health care, often with different monikers, the "decade of health information technology"[1] is upon us. Federal, state, and local governments and private sector initiatives have mushroomed to the point that the goal of EHR is becoming commonplace for nearly every healthcare organization. Although the Institute of Medicine (IOM) conducted a patient record study in the mid-1980s,[2] it was not until the IOM released its patient safety studies[3, 4, 5] that the need for health information technology was as acutely recognized. Today, the goal is to deliver consumer-centric and information-rich health care.

In the past, separate clinical departments in hospitals or specialty physicians primarily designed and installed clinical information systems. Oncology may have wanted a clinical system to support research. Pediatricians may have wanted to better track patient's immunizations. Endocrinologists may have found information technology to be helpful in managing chronic conditions. As a result, these groups developed many silos of highly sophisticated, clinical information systems. But these often remained the domain of the department or specialist. When the entire hospital, clinic, nursing facility, or other healthcare organization wanted to capture data from multiple sources and use it to support clinical decision-making at the point of care, they were left to kludge together information from disparate applications, use low-tech intermediaries for connectivity, and often supplement their decision-making with paper guidelines and visits to the Internet.

This book is not a substitute for experience in information system implementation. Rather, it is designed to

- provide an overview of EHR definition and migration path
- identify project management needs for the scope of planning represented by an EHR
- describe project planning for those new to using its principles
- offer suggestions for infrastructure preparedness unique to EHRs
- provide tools and techniques for process improvement and the behavioral changes needed to achieve those improvements

- describe the scope of EHR system build requirements
- impress upon users and technical support staff the importance of EHR testing
- offer strategies for pre-live conversion activities and training
- encourage the celebration of EHR success and lessons learned

Although there are differences in scope between types of healthcare facilities, this book's goal is to support any organization in its quest to carry out an EHR effectively and efficiently. Vendors will have highly detailed specifications and processes to which successful implementations must adhere. This book complements those specific instructions with strategies to deal primarily with the organizational, cultural, and change management factors of EHR implementation.

---

1. TG Thompson and DJ Brailer, *Framework for Strategic Action*, Progress Report (U.S. Department of Health and Human Services, Office of the National Coordinator for Health Information Technology: July 21, 2004).

2. Institute of Medicine, *The Computer-based Patient Record: An Essential Technology for Health Care*, (Washington, DC: National Academy Press, 1991, 1997).

3. Institute of Medicine, *To Err is Human: Building a Safer Health System* (Washington, DC: National Academy Press, 1999).

4. Institute of Medicine, *Crossing the Quality Chasm: A New Health System for the 21st Century* (Washington, DC: National Academy Press, 2001).

5. Institute of Medicine, *Patient Safety: Achieving a New Standard for Care* (Washington, DC: National Academies Press, 2004).

EHR Definition
and
Migration Path

CHAPTER 1

EHR Definition and Migration Path

Many healthcare professionals understand that electronic health records (EHR) are not systems to buy from the local vendor and install in a long weekend, or even over a course of a few weeks. Nor are they systems that can be set up "out of the box" or independently of other systems. Implementing an EHR is also more than just taking time or tailoring a system to your needs: It means truly engaging the user community in making a significant behavioral change.

The purpose of this chapter is to establish a common understanding of EHR. This material establishes the baseline upon which EHR selection, implementation, and benefits realization rests. Specifically, the chapter:

- defines EHR
- helps organizations understand potential user readiness for an EHR
- helps organizations understand financial and administrative readiness for an EHR (in the form of a return on investment (ROI) and value proposition)
- helps organizations understand the state of the art in EHR vendor offerings
- describes the need for a migration path toward an EHR
- points to standard functional descriptors for an EHR

EHR definition

Most industry observers define an EHR as a system that

- captures data from multiple sources
- is used as the primary source of information at the point of care
- provides evidence-based clinical decision support

Although it is a relatively straightforward statement, the definition of EHR is clearly more than hardware and software. An EHR system is also people, policies, and processes that define the way health care is delivered when supported by an EHR. In a way, an EHR is a mega-system: It requires that all sources of data in the healthcare organization be available to it. Users of the EHR are clinicians themselves. They are expected to use the system as they care for patients. In fact, as the primary source of information to care for patients, the EHR supplements clinician memory. The EHR also complements clinician knowledge by providing decision support. Clinicians interact directly with the system that supports their ability to tap a broad array of information and knowledge—to do what is right for the patient. Administrative, operational, and financial staff also use the EHR to further support patient care activities.

An EHR system, such as the one depicted in the model in Figure 1.1, depends on the presence of many factors. Whether the EHR is carried out in a hospital with many source systems or in a physician office with few source systems, among the most important factors—and the most unique to EHRs—are true system interoperability, data comparability, data quality, knowledge representation, and clinician adoption of process changes.

| Figure 1.1 | EHR model |

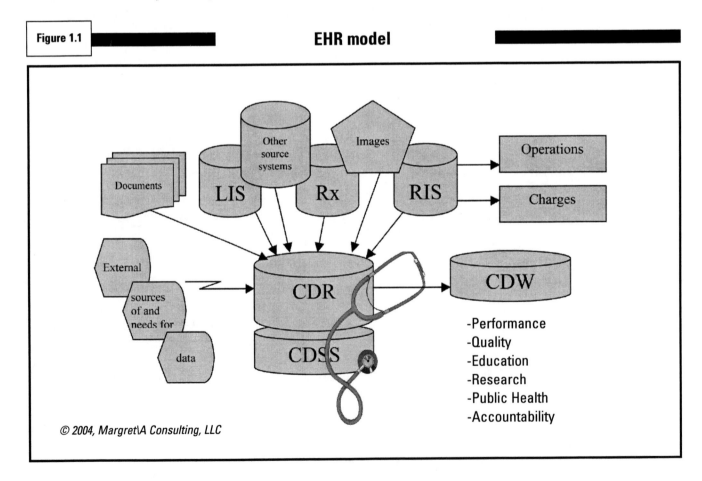

© 2004, Margret\A Consulting, LLC

System interoperability

All data needed to serve as the primary source of information must be available in electronic form for an EHR. Hence, all diagnostic studies results must be generated by information systems. Data captured on intake, during history-taking, and during physical examination must be in electronic form. Images that come from various medical devices must be put in a digital form.

In addition, the system must integrate data from all sources across applications. For an EHR to be used as the primary source of information, a user cannot be expected to go in and out of multiple applications to get bits and pieces of the total picture. Interoperability between applications contributes to the computer's ability to process data from the multiple sources into useful information.

- Basic interoperability refers to the ability of one information system to pass data to another.

- Functional interoperability is even more important. When passing data from one system to another, each system must understand the function or purpose of the data. Functional interoperability requires conformance to "message format standards," such as HL7, DICOM, NCPDP, IEEE, and others.

But even more than the ability to pass data from one application to the next, there needs to be the capability to manage large quantities of data in many ways. Typically, a clinical data repository (CDR) is used to pool data for such data management. Various other computational software systems or clinical decision support systems (CDSS) are then used to process the data in the repository or draw data into a clinical data warehouse (CDW) for further analysis. The end result is the ability, for example, to trend lab values against medications administered and simultaneously review an image of a cardiogram, or develop a new practice guideline based on evidence of actual results.

In an ideal system, data from other providers, patients themselves, pharmacies and pharmacy benefits managers, and other sources would be incorporated into an EHR. This is a broader view than most healthcare organizations today have for the EHR. Yet, this view is being supported within the context of a national health information infrastructure (NHII) and the regional health information organizations (RHIO) just starting to be formed. These structures are initially connecting a hospital and the providers affiliated with the hospital. Later they may connect pharmacies and other providers within a referral network. Even beyond that, there may be connectivity with payers to better support claims processing, eligibility, care management, disease management, and other functions. Ultimately, a NHII supports population health.

Data comparability and data quality

Data needed to support clinical decision-making in an EHR must be structured and codified. There also must be formal processes in place to ensure data quality. Documents containing handwritten notes that are scanned into a computer make information accessible, but the data contained in these documents are not structured or codified, and therefore cannot be processed by the computer. Document imaging may be needed to round out the full complement of information available, but this process does not support extensive interactive use of information technology. Computer systems that capture speech, handwriting, keyboard entry, or other forms of narrative data entry make the data that are accessible more legible but not necessarily easier to process. (Although document imaging, speech, handwriting, and keyboard all have the capability of producing discrete data when used with structured templates or indexing, many "EHR systems" today use these input processes primarily to collect an image of data or a narrative stream of text.)

To present alerts, reminders, prompts, logical branching, trends, and other value-added data, the original data must be discrete and unambiguous. It must also be accurate, precise, complete, and non-repudiated. A simple example is the erroneous result of comparing something measured in inches to something measured in centimeters. To achieve discrete and unambiguous data and promote data quality, there needs to be a common language, where each term has a precise meaning. In the past, information system vendors used internal data dictionaries, tables, and proprietary code sets to process data within their own systems. However, once data from applications supported by other vendors are put into a data repository, you need an overarching standard language. Clinical vocabularies, such as the Systematized Nomenclature of Medicine (SNOMED) for general medical and nursing terms, Logical Observations Identifiers Names and Codes (LOINC) for lab and other diagnostic studies results, RxNorm for clinical drugs, and others are used to achieve semantic interoperability. Semantic interoperability refers to the ability of a system to exchange data with another system where the meaning of data is also supported. Differences in types of interoperability are illustrated in Figure 1.2.

Figure 1.2

Interoperability

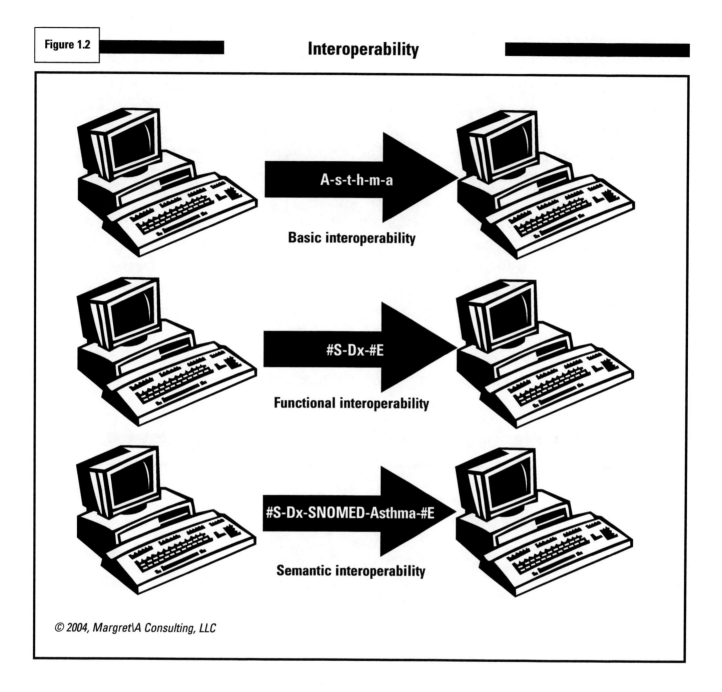

A-s-t-h-m-a

Basic interoperability

#S-Dx-#E

Functional interoperability

#S-Dx-SNOMED-Asthma-#E

Semantic interoperability

© 2004, Margret\A Consulting, LLC

Knowledge representation

Designers, implementers, and users must thoroughly understand the capabilities of information technology and information requirements of users to develop the means to capture quality data, convert the data to useful information, combine information from various sources to represent knowledge in clinical decision support, and provide such support when, and only when, needed. Figure 1.3 illustrates the data—information—knowledge continuum.

Many EHR vendors offer support for the knowledge continuum by way of structured templates, starter sets of clinical decision support rules, commonly available practice guidelines, report writers, and other tools. At a minimum, potential users must review them to determine whether they are acceptable. They may need to be modified to fit unique circumstances and they often need to be tailored to individual users and usage conditions. For example, a teaching hospital may need more frequent reminders and access to knowledge sources. Primary care physicians like to have structured templates and prompts, as well as access to the most current medical knowledge and patient's health plan formulary. Specialists frequently want alerts only when there is a serious potential contraindication, but they also want a concise summary of the patient's current health status and medications.

Figure 1.3	Data-information-knowledge continuum

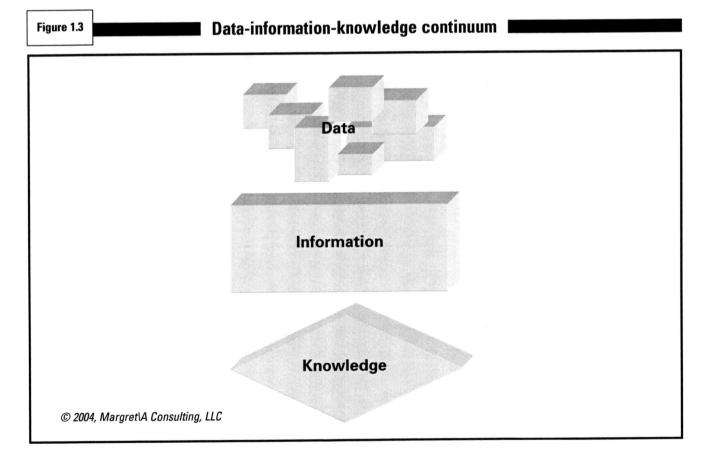

© 2004, Margret\A Consulting, LLC

Clinician adoption of process changes

Clinicians themselves are the key to achieving success with an EHR. This requires a significant level of process change, workflow redesign, and flexibility. Introducing such a significant level of change is nearly akin to asking humans to start writing with their feet or walking with their hands—feasible if they lose their hands or feet, but generally not something they'd take on voluntarily. The incentive in the case of the EHR must be of such value that the change is accepted voluntarily. Figure 1.4 explains why information systems need to produce value for clinicians.

Figure 1.4	EHR value example

A good example of the potential for value is computerized provider order entry (CPOE) systems, with which some hospitals have had good success and others have not.

Today's ordering practice is for a provider to handwrite an order, give it to a clerk who enters it into a computer, and have the computer disperse the instructions to the various departments that need to carry out the ordered procedures. If there are any questions about any of the instructions, the destination department calls the nursing unit. If the nursing unit cannot answer, the provider is contacted.

A basic CPOE system essentially turns the provider into a clerk. Even the suggestion that the order will be improved because the provider's intent will be clear is not necessarily valid, because, in the new position, a provider can just as easily key in an error or incomplete order.

But if the CPOE system were designed to capture structured data and run that data through clinical algorithms that would alert providers to contraindications, prompt for additional information, or remind them about duplicate procedures, there begins to be value to the provider.

Still, the true value often is not recognized, partly because more complete (order) documentation may take a bit longer to effect. Another part of the reason is that the value in CPOE tends to be downstream. Value (of CPOE) is often achieved through

- fewer calls and other interruptions after the order has been submitted
- more complete and correct orders, which ensure quality health

EHR readiness

Although most organizations have a vision of an EHR that is relatively consistent throughout the industry, deploying that vision has been difficult. User resistance, cost and ROI concerns, and vendor capability issues have gotten in the way.

People and processes

Cost and ROI concerns are often articulated as the main reasons for not acquiring an EHR, but an underlying factor of concern is resistance from potential users. Clinicians should use EHR systems at the point of care, but if they don't adopt it, the system will not achieve its intended benefits. And without achieving benefits, there is no reason to make the investment.

It is important to note that the term "clinicians" refers to all clinical users of the system, including physicians (whether employed or affiliated), nurses, pharmacists, laboratorians, therapists, and others. But in addition to clinicians, you must consider all other potential users. In fact, EHR systems that do not effectively support charge capture, reimbursement coding, release of information, reporting, and other functions as applicable to the type of healthcare organization are just as much at risk for failure as those that do not address clinician needs.

Although it is possible to mandate use of an information system for the employees to remain employed or for the medical staff to retain privileges, most healthcare organizations do not find this an effective way to set up an EHR. Factors that don't contribute to success of an EHR include disinterested, fearful, or antagonist physicians; ill-prepared staff; poor system design; and an unsupportive culture. Instead, people will find ways to work around it, won't adhere to new protocols, and will constantly demand changes that return processes to their manual form.

Preparing people to adopt new processes is potentially the most important factor in implementing an EHR—and one that is often overlooked or given short shrift. Some ways to assess readiness and prepare people are outlined in Figure 1.5.

| Figure 1.5 | **People and process readiness and preparation** |

Readiness indicators	Preparation
Expressed antagonism toward or lack of interest in EHR by physicians	Use physician specialty society information to promote EHR as becoming the standard of practice and care.
Fear of change by physicians	Offer clinical messaging, a provider portal, and other electronic forms of communication to illustrate value.
Concerns about cost and ROI by affiliated physicians and administration	Recommend vendor demos, attendance at conferences, and review of material that illustrates peer adoption and value.
Disinterest on the part of nurses and nursing personnel	Establish a migration path that introduces information technology step-by-step to overcome their biggest concerns and demonstrate patient safety.
Concerns expressed about the ability to perform nursing duties	This is often an expression of fear over learning to use a computer, where nurses typically have had the least exposure. Institute computer training courses that show (anyone) how to use navigational devices, what a browser is, how to troubleshoot problems, and how to enter and retrieve data. These training courses can be effective even when they address "fun" activities.
Ancillary departments having difficulty implementing new systems	Engage department staff in studying processes and offering their own improvements as buy-in for change. Establish expectations as part of acquiring new systems.
Therapists and other specialists who want "specialty" systems	Help them define their specific requirements and evaluate generic systems against them. Ensure that their special needs will be met to the extent reasonable.
Financial and administrative personnel who recommend bridge technology over EHR systems	Although bridge technology can be effective and may be an important part of a migration path, be aware that such interest may be based on concern about adoption and fear of losing jobs. Engage these personnel as integral parts of the EHR steering committee so they develop new skills and see themselves in new roles.

© 2004, Margret\A Consulting, LLC

Cost and ROI

As noted, cost and ROI are the most commonly articulated reasons for not acquiring an EHR. Realistically, organizations must address cost and ROI as significant issues. Not only must organizations find funds to pay for the EHR, but if managers begin to resent that EHRs aren't providing value, their negative attitudes may spill over to the users.

As a first step to addressing cost and ROI of EHR systems, healthcare organizations should take a critical look at what their processes cost today, where process and quality improvements are most important, and how they can structure a migration path toward an EHR to make smart investments over time.

Where most other industries are well-entrenched in computing unit costs for manufactured items or even service delivery, health care has never really been able to determine its unit costs. Part of the issue has been the high degree of variability in the human condition. Another important factor is the lack of incentives in the U.S. reimbursement process to perform well. In a fee-for-service environment, revenue increases when patients are sick and more services are provided. There is no incentive, other than ethical and moral, to improve care, so while care may not suffer to the extent suggested by this model because of ethical and moral principles, improvements in productivity have rarely seemed important. In a managed care environment, choice and access to services are restricted. As a result, providers are tentative and patients often settle for less than optimal health.

Normal economic principles simply do not apply to the way health care is structured in the United States. As a result, any attempt to conduct a cost/benefit analysis is extremely difficult. But many healthcare organizations are recognizing that change is in the wind. Third-party payers and the government are starting to offer pay-for-performance models and other incentive programs. Doing more with less has reached the breaking point. Executives and boards are also recognizing that a benefits portfolio is as important—if not more important—than a solely financial ROI.

A benefits portfolio should include cost savings, revenue increases, productivity improvement, patient safety, healthcare quality, and provider/patient satisfaction. Each of the portfolio components in turn moves the equation closer to ROI.

Cost savings

Although clearly a contribution to ROI, cost savings primarily accrue from administrative and operational factors associated with the EHR. For example, eliminating transcription costs is feasible if physicians perform all data entry directly at the point of care and the system itself generates summaries.

Some clerical staff, supplies, and archival expense reduction may be possible in chart filing and re-trieval functions for health information management (HIM) and patient financial services (PFS) areas. Organizations may reduce coding costs if the system generates codes from clinical documentation (pri-marily seen in physician office EHR systems, emergency departments, and outpatient areas). Inventory cost savings may be possible in various departments where EHR functionality (e.g., pharmacy invento-ry through a single formulary) can manage efficient use of inventory. Reductions in length of stay and cost of duplicate services through information availability are very likely.

However, make sure you critically appraise cost savings in staff reduction. There are some staff reduc-tions that are feasible. For example, overtime can sometimes be reduced or eliminated when charting does not have to extend beyond a shift. You may reduce recruitment/retention costs if the EHR system provides staff satisfaction. Most projected staffing reductions, however, are productivity improvements that allow for better quality of service. Furthermore, organizations must balance the cost savings they gain from other reductions against the new positions needed to maintain the EHR system.

Revenue increases

Increased revenue may result from EHR systems supporting enhanced documentation for charge capture and coding (especially in physician offices where down coding is commonplace). Some EHR systems improve productivity to the point where organizations (especially in physician offices) can reduce length of stay, see additional patients, or allow time for greater follow up with patients so they will return for more services. Pay-for-performance and other incentives for adopting EHR systems that contribute to patient safety and quality care can enhance revenue. Some organizations (especially hospitals) that have successfully implemented EHR systems are selling consulting services/hosting data centers.

Organizations often need to be creative to realize enhanced revenue from EHR systems. Take care when creating a message about EHR system benefits. It's important to make patients and their employers aware of EHRs to gain their support. However, the message must support the idea that the standard of practice is moving forward, rather than the misconception that EHRs are needed to fix the standard of practice.

Productivity improvement

Users may think that the time it takes to document in an EHR is longer than scrawling a progress note, scribbling an order, or placing a dot on a vital signs sheet—and in fact, if organizations were to perform time and motion studies, the time an entry takes may actually be several seconds longer in an EHR system. Seconds do add up to minutes and even hours. However, overall productivity improvements can be great from EHR systems because they can eliminate rework, errors, and, as previously noted, downstream time-wasters such as the following:

- Where did I put that scrap of paper on which I wrote the blood pressure?
- Did I use the napkin with the reminder written on it for cleaning up a spill?
- I better check the meds cart to see if I gave the med.
- In my haste, I used an unapproved abbreviation and have to respond to a telephone call as to its meaning.
- I forgot to give Mr. Andrews his meds at the appointed time, and now I have to check on the appropriate dose to give two hours later.

Every potential EHR user can identify many time-wasters where the EHR can make a difference. But the key to improvements is the sophistication of the systems and acceptance of new processes. Productivity improvements can mean more time caring for patients, which conceivably could lead to reduced lengths of stay, reduced errors, and increased patient satisfaction, which does translate into financial benefits.

Patient safety

Due to increased interest from the media and public press, patient safety is perhaps the biggest impetus for adopting EHR right now.

Just as healthcare organizations do not calculate their unit cost of services, they have often not captured patient safety information accurately. Most users do not believe the extent to which patient safety issues exist today or how EHRs can overcome them until they start using the systems and recognize the difference. Something as seemingly simple as missing Mr. A's meds can be a real eye-opening experience the first time the user is prompted to administer the meds or offers dosing information if the prompt fails to result in action (e.g., when there is a true emergency drawing staff away from normal duties).

Although medication ordering and administration provide the biggest "bang for the buck" in patient safety, there are many other patient safety measures that EHRs supply. They prompt a nurse to ask a patient about when he or she ate a meal before a procedure. They provide protocols for when patients need restraints. Obviously, patient safety can ultimately translate into cost savings where there is the potential for uncompensated care to manage adverse events, lawsuits, or "bad press."

Healthcare quality

The line between improving patient safety and healthcare quality may be fuzzy, but overall, most healthcare professionals believe that improved quality is a significant benefit of EHR systems. An EHR may suggest a differential diagnosis that a house staff member hadn't considered. It may remind a specialist to inquire about the success of a patient's smoking cessation program and be an additional support mechanism. It can automatically generate reminders to patients about health maintenance needs. It can prompt a physician to encourage a potential candidate to participate in a clinical trial. All of these functions and many others have the potential for producing cost savings/revenue.

Organizations can also use data collected during patient care to study performance, identify further quality improvement opportunities, help educate providers and patients alike, contribute to clinical research, support public health, and provide accountability for work performed. Overall quality improvement helps an organization differentiate itself in the marketplace, recruit the best and the brightest, and attract favorable contracts.

Provider and patient satisfaction

Provider and patient satisfaction may be the factor that is farthest removed from directly contributing to ROI but can be extremely important.

Many clinicians are frustrated when charts are not available, when lab results are not accessible, when an x-ray film has been lost, when a medication history is incomplete, or when they have to spend numerous hours on the phone collecting information about a patient from other providers.

Patients, too, are frustrated by the level of repetition in relating their past medical history or reason for visit. They are embarrassed when, as an otherwise intelligent person, they forget the exact name of the medication they are taking. Patients become concerned when test results are not available and interim measures are offered to resolve a problem. In addition, patients are becoming much more knowledgeable about health conditions and treatment regimens and expect their providers to be at least as knowledgeable and hopefully more so.

There are many patients who have researched new drugs with which their physicians are not familiar or alternative treatment regimens about which their physicians do not have the latest information. Even if they are not inclined toward such research, patients use computers at work, use them to check out their own groceries at the store, and expect that pilots use computer-assisted technology to fly the planes they board. Patients and their families also are routinely advised to be alert to and actively engage in their care during hospitalization. Although this involvement is certainly important, having to remember to take one's own medication or relying on a family member for information while the patient is in a semi-comatose state should not be the expected standard of practice.

Value proposition

Suffice it to say, the benefits of EHRs are real, despite their high cost and inability to necessarily predict an exact payback period or internal rate of return (IRR) for the investment. But for organizations to realize the benefits, executives and boards must establish expectations that there will be benefits, take steps to recognize them, and celebrate them.

Few healthcare organizations establish quantifiable metrics that they target for EHR success. Fewer still conduct benefits realization studies after implementation—primarily because there are no baseline data, but also because the systems take a long time to set up, so there are many confounding variables as time goes on. As a result, most healthcare organizations really do not know whether the EHR system has made a difference or not. Because squeaky wheels speak the loudest, executives and boards may only hear the complaints rather than the compliments.

Executives and boards should not have to take it on faith that EHRs produce benefits. Although formal benefits realization studies may not be feasible, some measures of success are critical. They help to celebrate success and confirm their value, and identify areas that may need improvement if certain aspects of EHR haven't produced the intended benefits.

Vendor offerings

Organizations also must consider another aspect of readiness: whether vendor offerings are ready to support their vision of an EHR. Vendors operate under the law of supply and demand. Information system vendors supply systems healthcare organizations want to buy. To date, these systems have been financial, operational, and specific to a department or facility-type (e.g., small physician office, clinic, or home health).

Although the concept of EHR has been around for a long time, healthcare organizations have not truly been in the market for buying these systems until very recently. All of the elements of resistance—cost, clinician disinterest, and resistance to change—have been stumbling blocks to even looking for an EHR system. As a result, many vendors have not put the research and development (R&D) time and expense into creating comprehensive, interoperable, knowledge-based EHR systems.

As a result, when healthcare organizations go to market today to find an EHR system, they may find less than what they currently envision. Hospitals are in a particularly problematic situation because of the legacy systems they currently have. Very often, hospitals will have interfaced systems from multiple vendors. Such interfaces allow the exchange of information from one system to another, but users must move in and out of separate applications to perform different functions. Figure 1.6 represents a common scenario.

Figure 1.6 **Hospital interface scenario**

Community General Hospital purchased a financial system from a major hospital information system (HIS) vendor in the early 1970s. Over time, it acquired other departmental systems—some from this vendor and some from other vendors that met the needs of the respective departments better. Some systems were interfaced to exchange demographic data.

When an order entry system from the HIS vendor was acquired in the late 1980s, interfaces were created to send the data to the departmental systems designated to receive orders where they existed and that were capable of having interfaces created. For other departments, paper order forms were written and sent through courier. The pharmacy was sent a facsimile of medication orders for patient safety purposes. Although laboratory results could be viewed by logging onto the laboratory information system, few used this feature because results were always printed.

Over time, the legacy systems were sunsetted by the vendor or found inadequate to meet emerging needs. As this occurred, departments went to market without regard to interoperability. In addition, many of these systems did not provide remote access, which was becoming of interest to the physicians in the community. To overcome these issues, the hospital purchased a viewer from its HIS vendor, where intra-organization and inter-organization access to lab results and dictated reports could be provided.

Recognizing the importance of information access to productivity where the small community struggled to retain clinical staff and recruit qualified physicians while its population aged and diminished in size, the hospital acquired a document imaging system in the mid-1990s. Some of the ancillary department systems could produce a computer output to laser disk (COLD) feed to the document management system. HIM department staff scanned other documents (not including nursing notes).

The document management system, however, was not compatible with the main HIS vendor's financial and administrative system so there was no connectivity with order entry or charge capture. Still, the hospital found the document management system useful, even though it had to use a separate terminal to view documents to check on charges or print information for claims attachments. The HIM department's

Figure 1.6 **Hospital interface scenario (cont.)**

encoder was not compatible with the system, although staff also found it helpful to use the document imaging system for release of information functions. Clinicians could retrieve scanned documents or COLD fed results from the document management system from their offices, although they rarely did so because not all documents were sufficiently indexed to find them rapidly and it was generally easier to call the hospital and have the document faxed. With the advent of patient safety concerns and interest in building a stronger community network, the hospital and physician community decided it was time to investigate an EHR. Their vision was sophisticated: They wanted a system that would serve each type of need, be fully compatible and interoperable, and provide clinical decision support.

Unfortunately, when they went to market, they found the EHR offered by the hospital's original HIS vendor to be inadequate. None of the physician office EHR vendors they looked at were capable of supporting a variety of sizes of offices or a hospital as a whole. At this point, they were faced with the potential for a massive overhaul of their systems, buying a repository and attempting to build their own EHR, or continuing to play the waiting game while hopefully upgrading and implementing new systems along a migration path that would ultimately lead them to being ready when their primary vendor was ready.

Although not every hospital has the mix of technology described in the scenario in Figure 1.6, many are still looking to their existing vendors to support more comprehensive EHR functionality. Many hospitals are still in the early stages of a migration path, building out their source systems. Others are actually beginning to consider major revamping of their existing systems and, in some cases, total replacement. A few hospitals are on the cutting edge of EHRs and have partnered with vendors for further development.

Physician offices and other types of healthcare organizations may have a somewhat easier time in acquiring an EHR that meet their needs. They often have not yet made a major investment in feeder systems or even the technical infrastructure to support an EHR. When they go to market, they are essentially starting from scratch and can buy an integrated system from one vendor that provides billing, practice management, and EHR functionality. Even this scenario, however, is changing as providers are rapidly becoming interested in connecting with other providers to share referral information and, to a lesser extent, to take advantage of best practices and research opportunities. Physicians in a community may find that one or two offices have already made separate and disparate purchases, and none offer easy exchange of information among the providers or with the hospital.

Vendors will clearly need to step up their R&D efforts, but the industry can only expect them to do so when the demand is present and real. To some extent, this may be a "chicken and egg" situation. But more and more healthcare organizations are moving to technology such as document imaging, speech dictation, provider portals, clinical messaging, and others to bridge the gaps. As a result of this movement, vendors are starting to ramp up to more comprehensive systems.

EHR migration path

As suggested earlier in this chapter, there are many benefits and many barriers to EHR adoption. In general, organizations that have developed strategic plans for information technology or a proactive EHR migration path are in better shape than their counterparts who have taken a more reactive position. A migration path is most helpful if it identifies the generic types of functions the organization needs it to perform, identifies the technology to carry out those functions, and identifies the benefits expected.

Figure 1.7 offers a model of a migration path that healthcare organizations may find useful. The first two functions, data access and work flow, are often accomplished through existing systems that are interoperable or through the adoption of bridge technology. The biggest benefit is data availability. The next two functions, documentation and decision support, represent the biggest hurdles to be overcome—clinician resistance and cost. Unfortunately, these two functions are generally inseparable. As suggested by the scenario in Figure 1.4, it is difficult to get clinicians to document in an information system without value being returned to them. These functions represent the primary purpose of the EHR. The last function, predictive modeling, is a function that some organizations may be able to integrate within others or that other organizations may take a very long time to accomplish.

The migration path in Figure 1.7 is not intended to be an "answer" for everyone. Experts tend to agree on the functionality path and the benefits it will generate, but there are many technologies to achieve the various functions and benefits.

Figure 1.7 **EHR migration path**

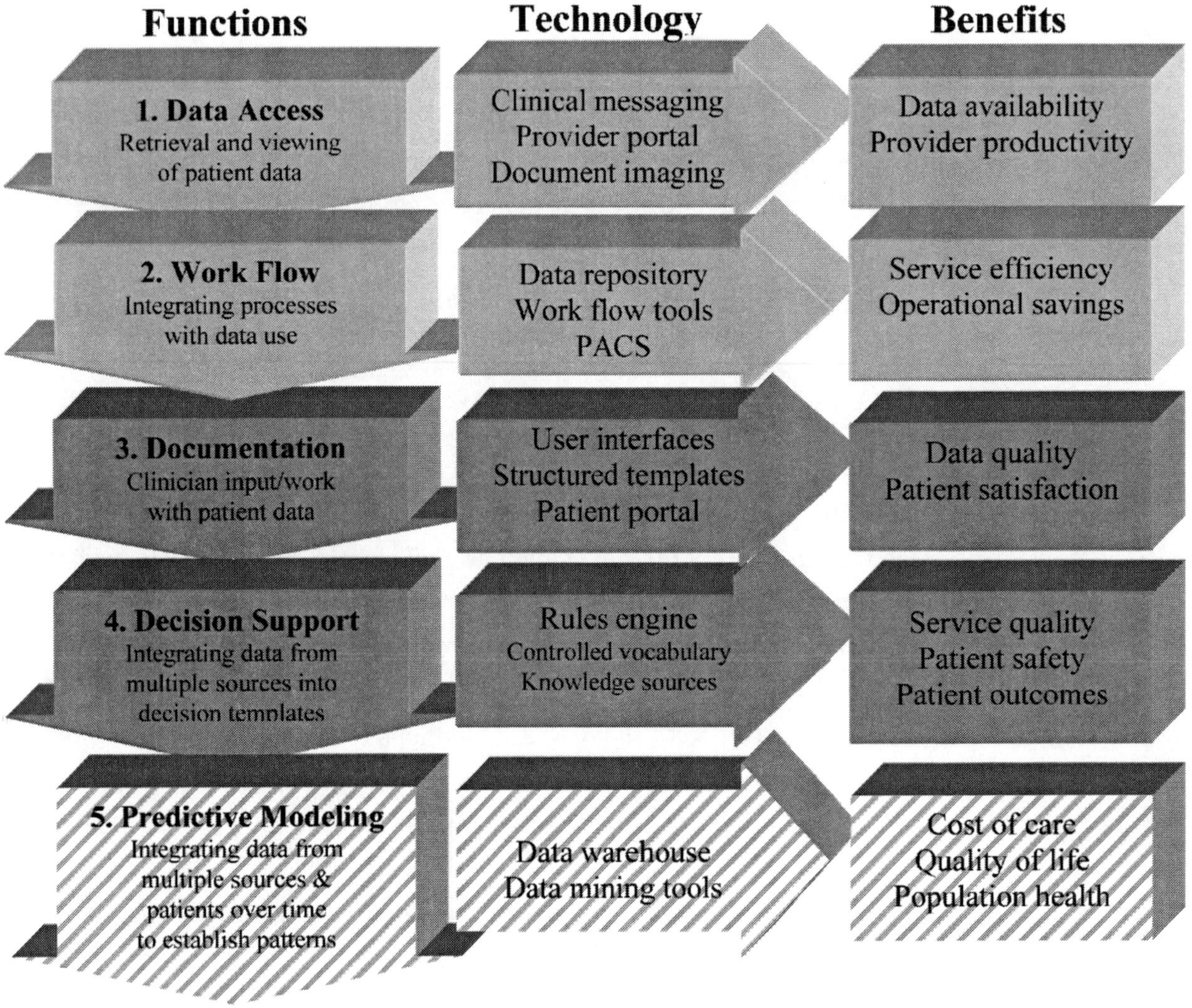

Functions

1. Data Access
Retrieval and viewing
of patient data

2. Work Flow
Integrating processes
with data use

3. Documentation
Clinician input/work
with patient data

4. Decision Support
Integrating data from
multiple sources into
decision templates

5. Predictive Modeling
Integrating data from
multiple sources &
patients over time
to establish patterns

Technology

Clinical messaging
Provider portal
Document imaging

Data repository
Work flow tools
PACS

User interfaces
Structured templates
Patient portal

Rules engine
Controlled vocabulary
Knowledge sources

Data warehouse
Data mining tools

Benefits

Data availability
Provider productivity

Service efficiency
Operational savings

Data quality
Patient satisfaction

Service quality
Patient safety
Patient outcomes

Cost of care
Quality of life
Population health

© 2004, Margret\A Consulting, LLC

HL7 EHR functional descriptors

Another approach to plotting a migration path is to use the EHR functional descriptors as adopted by Health Level Seven (HL7) as a draft standard for trial use (DSTU). This model of the functional descriptors is illustrated in Figure 1.8.

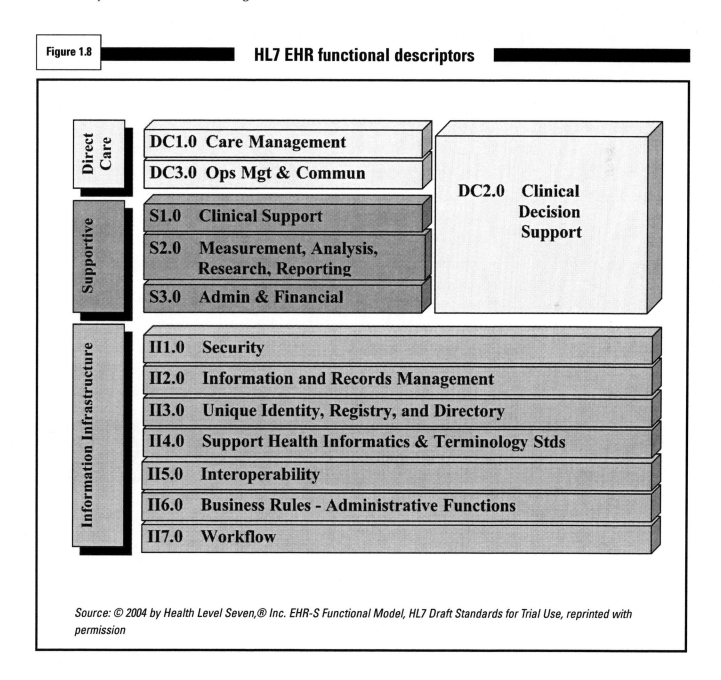

Figure 1.8 — **HL7 EHR functional descriptors**

Direct Care
- DC1.0 Care Management
- DC3.0 Ops Mgt & Commun

Supportive
- S1.0 Clinical Support
- S2.0 Measurement, Analysis, Research, Reporting
- S3.0 Admin & Financial

DC2.0 Clinical Decision Support

Information Infrastructure
- II1.0 Security
- II2.0 Information and Records Management
- II3.0 Unique Identity, Registry, and Directory
- II4.0 Support Health Informatics & Terminology Stds
- II5.0 Interoperability
- II6.0 Business Rules - Administrative Functions
- II7.0 Workflow

Source: © 2004 by Health Level Seven,® Inc. EHR-S Functional Model, HL7 Draft Standards for Trial Use, reprinted with permission

In the model, the information infrastructure functions and lower levels of each of the supportive and direct care functional categories represent functions equivalent to data access and work flow in the Figure 1.7 migration path. Most organizations must face the challenge of adopting technology to provide further supportive functionality, direct care management, and clinical decision support (represented as documentation and decision support in Figure 1.7's migration path). The HL7 functional descriptors model does not extend beyond the enterprise as suggested by the benefits of predictive modeling in the Figure 1.7 migration path, although many of the functions employed through data warehouses and data mining tools would address measurement, analysis, research, and reporting. The full HL7 DSTU is available from *www.hl7.org*. Although the press release that accompanied the announcement of the standard indicates that the model would "provide a common language for the provider community to help guide their planning, acquisition, and transition to electronic systems, and . . . facilitate a more effective dialogue between providers and vendors," HL7 also notes that the model is not a conformance tool. Furthermore, it describes a gradual compliance: "It is important to note that compliance with the standard does not mean that every function of the model be addressed by every vendor immediately."

The press release further notes that some functions are visionary, some are more important to one care setting than to another, and the standard is voluntary. "Vendors can choose which of the EHR functions they include in their products and by what timeline they will include them."[1] Figure 1.9 is a sample functional statement from the DSTU.

| Figure 1.9 | **HL7 sample functionality statement** | |

ID	Formative ballot content		Functional description	See also	Rationale	Citation
	Function name	Function statement				
DC.1.1.3.3	Manage allergy and adverse reaction list	Create and maintain patient-specific allergies and reactions	Allergens and substances are identified and coded (whenever possible) and the list is managed over time. All pertinent dates, including patient-reported events, are stored and the description of the patient allergy and reaction is modifiable over time. The entire allergy history, including reaction, for any allergen is viewable.		Supports delivery of effective healthcare. Facilitates management of chronic conditions.	

Source: Copyright 2004 by Health Level Seven,® Inc. EHR-S Functional Model, HL7 Draft Standards for Trial Use, reprinted with permission.

EHR vision

The EHR definition, readiness assessment, migration path, and functional descriptors discussed in this chapter should provide anyone embarking on an EHR implementation with a solid understanding of what an EHR is and the extent to which it is being implemented in the healthcare organization.

This chapter highlights the complexity of an EHR, its differences from other systems implemented in healthcare organizations, and the mission criticality of the system. Understanding of these elements will hold any implementation team member, super user, project manager, or analyst in good stead as the implementation actually occurs. Unlike any other information system, the EHR has the most direct link to patient care.

End notes

1. Health Level Seven, Inc., Press Release (March 11, 2004).

CHAPTER 2

EHR System Acquisition

CHAPTER 2

EHR System Acquisition

In addition to creating a vision of an EHR and migration path toward that goal, a healthcare organization must develop a request for proposal (RFP), select a vendor, and negotiate a contract to acquire and implement the EHR. Although these functions precede implementation, there are important factors inherent in them that organizations must understand. This chapter

- compares the purposes and processes associated with a selection committee and a project steering committee
- describes an RFP and how to identify and define EHR functional requirements
- outlines the vendor selection process in which organizations can determine and validate the existence of EHR functionality support in a vendor product
- identifies contract negotiation components that directly relate to successful implementation of EHR

Selection committee

Form an EHR selection committee either at the point your organization decides to begin its vendor selection or during the visioning and migration path planning stage. The EHR selection committee must be interdisciplinary and interdepartmental. Figure 2.1 on the following page lists typical members of such a committee.

In large organizations, there may be subcommittees of the selection committee that address various aspects of the selection process. For example, there may be a physician advisory committee, a nursing advisory committee, and a finance committee.

Figure 2.1	EHR selection committee

Membership	Purpose
Chief operating officer	Executive sponsor
Medical director of information systems, medical informaticist	Will be responsible for coordinating physician EHR processes
Representative of affiliated medical staff	Liaison to physician community
Representative physician from hospitalist, intensivist, or other employed physician, if applicable	Will be among primary physician users
Representative member of house staff, if applicable	Will be among primary physician users
Nurse informaticist	Will be responsible for coordinating nursing EHR processes
Representative nurse(s) and unit clerk	Will be among primary nursing users
Health information management professional	Provides primary support for information management functions
Representative from patient financial services	Needs to ensure charge capture and other financial functions are integrated with EHR
Chief information officer	Provides primary support for information technology functions
Representatives from major ancillary departments impacted by EHR	Ensures interoperability of processes
For example: Pharmacy, Laboratory, Radiology, Others	Consultant
	Legal counsel
	Chief financial officer
Others as needed:	Quality, compliance, risk managers
	Human resources/labor relations
	Others

Steering/project management committee

Whatever the committee's size and scope, it usually exists throughout the entire process and then disbands. Some members may then participate on a steering committee or EHR selection project management committee that supports the EHR implementation. Frequently, there is a mix of some former selection committee members and new members who are more focused on project management, process improvement, and installation, testing, training, or benefits realization.

Again, in large organizations, there may be several subcommittees or teams. These teams will perform the actual infrastructure preparation, process improvement planning, and system build, testing, training, and benefits realization.

Request for proposal

The first task for the selection committee is to clearly articulate the healthcare organization's desired functionality and prepare an RFP. The HL7 EHR Functional Descriptors Draft Standard for Trial Use (DSTU) can provide an excellent checklist to aid a healthcare organization in identifying the desired functions to match its EHR vision and for going to market for an EHR. This checklist is often included in an RFP.

RFP *outline of content*

An RFP can be a very large document. Most healthcare organizations continue to use a traditional RFP, especially for major systems purchases such as EHRs. The content of an RFP for an EHR is outlined in Figure 2.2 on p. 30.

Functional requirements specification

The functional requirements section of the RFP is the core description of what the buyer wants to buy. Although some parts of an RFP may be boilerplate for any major information system acquisition, the functional specifications are unique to an EHR system. This is the part of the process in which users typically are asked to contribute their thoughts. Although it serves to capture and compare information from various vendors about various products, the functional requirements also allow users to offer input, and the organization can capture the vision of an EHR on paper.

In addition to articulating the vision and desired specifications, this section serves as a checklist so the organization can understand what it is buying and, later, to evaluate its benefits. Although the functional requirements section can take different forms, the narrative and structured formats are the most common.

Figure 2.2 **RFP content outline**

I. Introduction and general instructions for response

II. Background information (of buyer)

- Goals and objectives for going to market
- Current systems in use
- Volumes and statistics
- Target timeline for decision and implementation

III. Vendor profile: Captures information on . . .

- Company contact
- Organization chart
- Personnel
- Corporate identity
- Corporate financial status
- System history
- System release methodology
- Future plans
- Field offices
- Client references
- User groups
- Legal and working relationships with other suppliers
- Pending litigation

IV. Functional requirements: Include . . .

- Functional specifications checklist
- Clarification needed on checklist (provides notes and supporting material)
- HIPAA and other regulatory requirements

Figure 2.2 ███████████ **RFP content outline (cont.)** ███████████

V. Technical requirements: Include . . .

- Infrastructure and communications network
- Hardware, peripherals, and network
- Operating system and application software
- Interfaces/connectivity requirements and capabilities
- User flexibility tools
- Response time
- Redundancy and recovery
- Database: administration and access
- Data security and rights of access
- Maintenance
    ‣ Hardware engineering support
    ‣ Software engineering support
    ‣ Estimate of hardware support to be provided by client
- Disaster recovery and support
- Environmental considerations
    ‣ Electrical
    ‣ Environmental requirements (air-conditioning, humidity control, etc.)
    ‣ Space
- Warranties and guarantees

VI. Implementation: Requires . . .

- Delivery schedule
- Implementation schedule
- System tailoring and table generation
- Acceptance test procedures
- Implementation approach
- General vendor support
- Issue resolution process

| Figure 2.2 | RFP content outline (cont.) |

VII. Training and documentation: Requires . . .

- Training programs included/available
- Required certifications
- Documentation, including implementation guidelines, installation instructions, source code, etc.

VIII. Contractual considerations: Requires . . .

- Proposal to be attached to the contract
- Specific contractual terms and conditions (if any)
- Standard contract to be attached
- Vendor contract acceptability

IX. Cost presentation (include explicit instructions for format and level of detail),
including directions to submit apart from above components.

© 2004, Margret\A Consulting, LLC

- Narrative formats require the vendor to respond to questions in a descriptive manner. For example, organizations might ask, "Please describe how your system provides a closed-loop medication process." The vendor should then describe how the process is achieved.

The advantage of this approach is that, if properly completed by the vendor, the description provides the buyers with a good understanding of how the system is intended to work. The major disadvantage for the buyer is that it is very difficult to identify objective criteria for assessing and comparing responses from vendors, especially since the quality and level of detail in the responses may vary greatly and do not necessarily reflect product capabilities. The major disadvantage for the vendor is the level of effort it takes to properly respond to each question. To compensate for the disadvantages, keep the number of questions short, addressing only the most important considerations of a system and those likely to represent the greatest differences among the vendors. This approach works best for buyers who are very knowledgeable about such systems and are comfortable working without strict guidelines for comparing responses between vendors.

- Structured formats include a detailed checklist of requirements to which vendors respond "yes," "no," or "to be developed," along with the option to provide additional information or explanation. More rigorous RFPs would require vendors to indicate the status of each requirement, using categories such as the following:

  - Generally available and installed in one or more client sites
  - Generally available and installed in one or more client sites, but not part of this proposal (perhaps it is part of a module the buyer did not express interest in buying)
  - Being used in one or more client sites, but not available for general release yet (i.e., in alpha/beta testing)
  - Planned for future release
  - Not available, but will develop for additional fee
  - Not available, no current plans to develop

It is not unusual for such checklists to exceed one thousand discrete questions, though many experts believe it makes sense to limit the number of questions to those that will most help differentiate vendors/products.

If your organization plans to use the HL7 EHR Functional Descriptors as a basis for functional requirements specifications, review them thoroughly, list all the ones you actually want, and add any specifications the vendor doesn't include. Although you may be tempted to ask whether the vendor is "compliant" with the HL7 EHR Functional Descriptors, you can't expect all vendors to have all functionality.

Vendor selection

Developing and submitting the RFP to vendors are just two steps in a well-defined and managed process to select an EHR. The goal of vendor selection should be to find the vendor with the best overall fit for your organization's needs. As noted in Chapter 1 under "Migration path and HL7 functional descriptors," EHR products mean different things to different people. It is unlikely that you'll find a product that meets absolutely all specifications. Although it's beneficial to find an EHR product that has most of the desired functions, it may not be a good choice if the vendor is on the verge of bankruptcy. View the process of vendor selection as passing the universe of vendors through a funnel, such as illustrated in Figure 2.3. To manage the vendor selection process, consider the following steps:

Figure 2.3	EHR vendor selection process

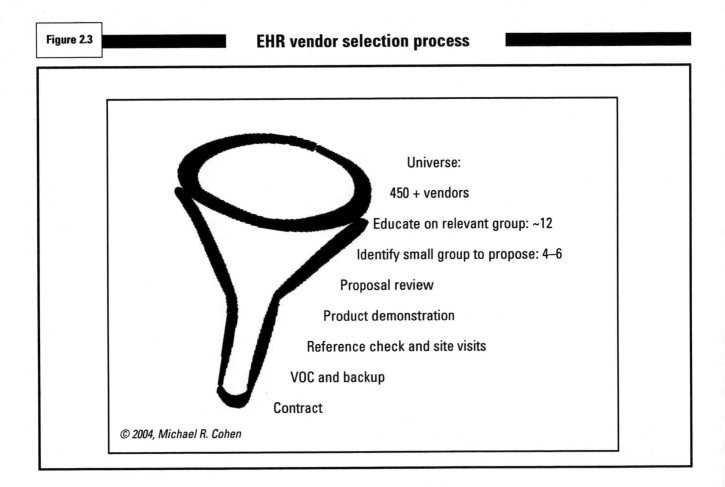

Universe:

450 + vendors

Educate on relevant group: ~12

Identify small group to propose: 4–6

Proposal review

Product demonstration

Reference check and site visits

VOC and backup

Contract

© 2004, Michael R. Cohen

Step one: Narrow the universe

Your first goal is to narrow the field to about 12 vendors to review for potentially sending an RFP. There are many EHR vendors (or those claiming to have EHR products)—far too many to whom your organization can realistically send RFPs. To narrow the field, look at the vendors' market characteristics, such as those listed in Figure 2.4.

Figure 2.4	EHR market characteristics

Characteristic indicators	Variables indicators
Type of organization for which EHR is supplied	IDN, hospital, ambulatory surgery center, clinic, physician office, home health agency, nursing facility, etc.
Size of organization for which EHR is supplied	Small, medium, large within the target type of organization
Geographic location for which EHR is supplied	International, national, regional concentrations
Key EHR functionality	Major modules, such as CPOE, patient portal, clinical decision support, clinical data warehouse, etc.
Method to deliver EHR functionality	In-house, remote hosted, application service provider (ASP)
Technology platform for EHR	Windows-based, UNIX-based, other
Relative costs of EHR	Expensive, moderate, inexpensive
Incumbent information systems vendors	Because interoperability is often (though not always) best achieved through buying from the same vendor, an organization's existing major vendor(s) generally should be considered

© 2004, Michael R. Cohen

You can find sources of information on market characteristics in professional journals and trade publications; professional organizations such as HIMSS, MGMA, AHIMA, specialty societies, etc.; trade shows, major industry events and award/recognition programs; information technology consultants; and networking with colleagues at other healthcare organizations. This can be labor-intensive, but it pays to narrow the field early. Limiting the field to about a dozen vendors is manageable—with more than that, the process will become unwieldy.

Step two: Narrow the field

Next, identify a handful (four to six) of vendors with whom you want to work during the RFP/buying process. Do not underestimate the effort saved and value of going to market with a manageable number of vendors. Not only does it reduce the time you will spend reviewing proposals, talking with vendors, etc., but also it allows you to spend quality time with each vendor. In return, the vendors will appreciate the smaller field of competitors. Because their chances of winning are better in a smaller field, they are more likely to devote the resources needed for the sales effort, resulting in better information and less frustration for your organization.

Most organizations develop a short list of key criteria that they use to narrow the field. This list of criteria is also often used for reviewing responses to the actual RFP. See Figure 2.5 for an example of criteria used for an EHR selection.

Figure 2.5	Relevant vendor criteria

- Key functionality
- Vendor viability to continue as a strong player in the market
- Vendor technical support
- Training support
- Implementation effort and approach
- Implementation support
- Technology/architecture
- Vision (R&D momentum)
- Integration
- Vendor's clinical culture
- Return on investment
- Cost relative to budget

© 2004, Margret\A Consulting, LLC

Many organizations do not include cost at this point. Cost can vary by configuration, delivery method, and other factors—all of which your organization can negotiate later in the process. A surrogate for cost might be return on investment (ROI). If other organizations have had positive results, it is very likely that the ROI is sufficient to support the investment.

Step three: Proposal review

Once you send the RFP to the small field of competitors, along with clear directions on how to respond and a reasonable and clearly articulated timeframe (about four weeks) for response, you must review the proposals your organization received. Some organizations refuse to consider late responses, suggesting that lateness reflects the vendor's business practices. Others will accept a late response if the vendor provides adequate and reasonable notice.

Reviewing vendor responses to the RFP is an educational process. You must analyze the vendors' feature and function capabilities, as well as other factors and attributes addressed in the RFP and defined in the selection criteria. Although the process should include an objective scoring and quantification of vendor responses, the scoring is just a means to an end. Numeric scores are meaningless if your organization hasn't taken the time to understand what the vendor is offering, hasn't identified questions and issues to present to the vendor, or is just beginning to develop personal opinions of how good a fit one vendor is compared to others. The proposal review is still only near the middle of the funnel.

Interestingly enough, as your organization moves to the next stage of narrowing the field, it will need less data to make informed choices. The selection committee will become more able to focus on the differences between vendors and concentrate on the factors that most impact the decision. It is not unusual, after going through all the steps of the process, to base the final decision on just a handful of most important differentiators. The end result of RFP response review should be some objective and quantifiable comparison of the vendors. If it is very obvious that certain vendors are not competitive, eliminate them from further consideration.

Step four: Product demonstrations

Product demonstrations provide your organization with the opportunity to see products much more closely, through a live "show and tell" process in which the vendor walks through the system and provides examples of various functions. Vendors will set up equipment at your location with their product either loaded on a local computer or connected to their remote host computer.

For a large organization, EHR product demonstrations can turn into a "vendor fair," which allows dozens of potential users from the organization to view the demos over the course of several days. If your organization chooses this method, you must carefully manage the process. Notify the vendors of your expectations, set ground rules about their contacting and "selling" throughout the organization, and have a solid agenda so that they have enough time to address each major area. Educate staff and set ground rules for them as well. A vendor will try to find a strong "inside salesperson" who will endorse its system. To avoid this scenario, make sure staff understand the risk of becoming a spokesperson for a particular vendor.

Explain to vendors you want them to bring to the EHR demo their "A team" of experienced personnel, including a senior marketing staff representative; a former user from a client; and a nurse, HIM professional, or other clinical professional; and ideally, a physician. These individuals typically make the best presenters for EHR systems since they can relate to potential user's needs and circumstances.

Develop demonstration scripts that outline what the vendor is supposed to show in each application area, such as using examples or scenarios from your organization. Using scripts keeps the buyer, rather than the vendor, in control of what is being presented. This assures your organization that vendors will address the most important areas, rather than only those the vendor believes are important—which will most likely coincide only with their product strengths. Keeping control of this process will also provide your organization with a more objective and "apples to apples" comparison of the vendors.

Step five: Reference checks and site visits

Your organization should have enough information at the end of product demonstrations to identify the best and the weakest. Ideally, your goal is to narrow the field to vendor finalists that have the best overall fit. To validate your decision, check references with each vendor's client base and with site visits.

Various members of the selection committee can participate in reference checking. The most powerful and meaningful reference checks are those performed on a peer-to-peer basis (e.g., clinician talking to clinician, IT staff talking to IT staff, etc.). You can use a standard questionnaire, such as the one provided in Figure 2.6, as a template that each team member can tailor to fit his or her needs.

Because reference checking, and the site visits that follow, may put your organization at odds with the bidding vendors, it is important to take control of the situation. For example, some vendors insist that potential buyers only contact an "approved list" of reference sites and only specific individuals within a site. They may even insist on arranging and joining the calls, claiming they want to minimize disruption to their current clients. And although there may be some merit to such a vendor-managed approach, it will also mean your organization will only receive the best references. It is equally important to contact mediocre and even bad references (every vendor of any size has at least one) in order to get a clearer picture of the vendor and any patterns. These references help identify pitfalls so your organization can develop contingency plans if you choose that vendor. However, finding these references may require some investigative work. One way to approach this is to ask for a list of all clients.

Figure 2.6   **Reference check information**

Questions indicators	Positive findings indicators	Negative findings indicators
1. Is the vendor's reference site similar to the buyer? What was the reference site's vision and expectations?		
2. What product/version was acquired? Is that the same as currently under consideration?		
3. How long did it take to implement the EHR? Was implementation on time and on budget?		
4. What is the general satisfaction level with the EHR? Is there full adoption? If not, why not?		
5. What are specific strengths and weaknesses of the EHR?		
6. What would the reference site do differently if going to market for an EHR all over again?		

© 2004, Michael R. Cohen

Another approach would be to contact those that have been supplied and ask them who they contacted for information. You can also try contacting those you know who have recently undertaken an EHR selection process and settled on another vendor and ask them why they chose the other vendor. Finally, you can join a list serve through your professional society and solicit contacts for organizations that have the products you are considering.

You should arrange site visits to vendor clients that are similar in nature to your organization and that use the vendor's EHR that is comparable to the one you intend to use. Note that this matching process can be a difficult and frustrating task. Often a vendor's installed base will have earlier versions of the product or a very different mix of source systems or organizational characteristics. In the end, you may have to compromise or make more than one site visit per vendor.

To make the most of the site visits, have a clear agenda and minimize vendor control to ensure an objective and unbiased view. Use your time at the client site to *observe the impact the* EHR *has on the organization*. Ask peers to demonstrate the use of the system and describe what improvements they have noted, what processes have been improved, or what evidence they have of improvements, etc. Don't ask the client site to conduct the same type of product demonstration as the vendor. Instead, tour the facility, talk with peers, and observe the impact of the system.

Invite several different types of future users to the visit. If the vendor insists on being present, have at least two or three people attend from the organization so at least one of them can slip away, observe, and talk to random users at the site. Use this time to verify the presence or absence of key product capabilities that are influencing your decision, such as getting hard evidence from the site visit host that the capabilities are real.

Step six: Vendor of choice and back-up determination

By the conclusion of the site visits, you should have sufficient information to make a decision on the vendor of choice (VOC), and perhaps the back up. In the perfect world, the "second place" vendor would be strong enough to be the VOC if you can't finalize an agreement with the "number one" vendor. Remember, if the process is working well, the selection team's final decision should boil down to a small number of items that truly differentiate the vendors. The members of the team need to think of the organization's best interests, not their own, when forming a consensus. In other words, in order to achieve strong integration and an EHR that truly works, some individuals may need to compromise their proprietary interests in favor of the best interests of the overall organization.

Step seven: Contract negotiation

Once you select your VOC, you'll begin contract negotiations or at least ask your organization's executive management for approval to move to that step.

The primary objective of contract negotiation is to clarify precisely what is and what isn't being acquired (whether the EHR is bought, leased, or otherwise acquired). Contract negotiation addresses the exact product (version, applications, modules, etc.), computer and network configurations, service levels, implementation effort, ongoing support, etc. This is much more difficult than first appears. Vendor packaging for EHR systems is so complex that it will take much discussion just to agree on what specific applications and modules your organization is acquiring. This process is compounded by a seemingly endless array of potential "add-ons," a myriad of options on how to implement the system, a vast array of file conversion tools to select from, etc. The technology layer requires agreement on equipment configuration, including precise number of devices, network requirements, back up, security options, etc. Although you should discuss these issues throughout the buying process, it all needs to come together in the form of a written contractual agreement.

The second objective of contract negotiation is to clearly understand obligations and requirements, not only financially, but also in terms of the organization's role in implementing and supporting the system. Contract negotiations are about much more than cost. In fact, there is a danger to placing too much emphasis on cost early in the negotiation process. First, many of the contract issues will have economic impact, making it very difficult for the vendor to know exactly where and to what to apply cost. Second, if you agree on a price too early, it makes it easy for the vendor to either refuse concessions on other issues or to reopen cost discussion. (See Figure 2.7 for a summary of issues you should address during contract negotiations.)

| Figure 2.7 | Contract negotiation issues |

Issue	Considerations
Product functionality	Product descriptions that were stated verbally or "promised" during the sales cycle will have no contractual validity unless they are in writing and attached to the contract. Many buyers are surprised that most contracts stipulate that what is bought is the product as defined in the vendor's product/user documentation. In other words, if capabilities are not adequately addressed in the manuals or added specifically to the contract, the vendor is not contractually obligated to deliver them. A painful but useful process is to have a team of users review the vendor documentation to validate understanding of what is being bought and supplement it with written responses from the vendor that are attached to the contract.
Cost and payment terms	Issues such as payment terms that are tied to performance can potentially be worth more than large price concessions because they nail down the vendor on performance. Agreement on the proper number of licenses, or seats, that being bought directly drives price, and can make cost look artificially low if it is discovered that not enough licenses were acquired for proper use of the system. Getting price protection for future purchases or for expanded use of the system can save many dollars down the line, as can limiting the size of annual increases for maintenance and support. As mentioned above, just about anything can have some economic impact on the vendor.

Figure 2.7 **Contract negotiation issues (cont.)**

Technical	Interfaces, system performance, uptime/downtime, response time, assurance of proper hardware/network configuration, etc., need to be fully explored and agreed upon.
Implementation	How the system is implemented will have as much impact on the true value of the system (and perhaps as much cost) as the product and vendor. It is wise to nail down the implementation approach and level of effort before signing the contract. Most vendors prefer to deal with implementation details after the contract is signed, but it is best to do pre-implementation planning concurrent with contract negotiation. At a minimum, this should define implementation phases, timing and milestones within phases, level of vendor support, internal level of effort (which will be measured in many people years of effort), and a preliminary project organization. Other implementation issues, such as assurances that vendor implementation staff will be fully qualified or having a right to review their backgrounds, are also fertile ground for discussion.
Other business issues	It is surprising how many other details will be noticed and addressed by a thorough review of the contract. This can be anything ranging from defining potential roles/limitations as a future "site visit host location" to incorporating HIPAA privacy concerns and business associate agreements.
Legal issues	It is critical for an EHR contract to be reviewed by an attorney knowledgeable in the laws and contracts surrounding information systems. Remember, this system is to be used directly by staff and affiliates, and it directly impacts patient care. There must be adequate legal safeguards and protections against false claims, indemnification, etc.

A few other guiding principles to successful EHR system negotiation include the following:

- Obtaining a "performance based" contract—an EHR is a solution to important clinical and business needs, not just a set of software programs and days of effort to help install it.
- Finding solutions that will please both your organization and vendor whenever possible.
- Understanding your vendor's needs and style at the negotiation table.
- Identifying and resisting (or creating leverage from) closing tactics.
- Remaining firm, but being reasonable and honest.
- Getting the issues on the table early. A comprehensive letter outlining all known issues shared with the vendor helps establish credibility, and helps both sides better understand how to prepare.
- Reading the details of the contract carefully.

Readiness for project planning

Once you've resolved the devilish details, you can begin actual implementation activities. As this chapter has illustrated, however, there is great value in knowing about potential pitfalls or weaknesses in advance. It is also essential that the implementation process follow the contractual requirements, or the contract could be put at risk.

C H A P T E R   3

Project Planning and Managing

CHAPTER 3

Project Planning and Managing

Once the ink is dry on the EHR contract, it's time to start planning the implementation process in detail. When EHR implementations fail, it is often due to inadequate project planning and management. The complexity of an EHR system and its multiple touch points make it particularly difficult to implement. In addition, the EHR system impacts people who in many cases are not currently computer users. If a governance structure is not already in place, this is the time to create one. Designate someone to manage the project timeline, budget, and scope; develop a detailed plan of action; establish an issue resolution process; and plan for ongoing maintenance and upgrading. Specifically, this chapter

- offers suggestions for effective project governance
- describes the roles and responsibilities for the project manager
- urges you to approach EHR implementation from a team perspective
- provides a detailed plan of attack for preparing the infrastructure, redesigning work flow and processes, conducting "system build," testing, converting, training, and celebrating "go live"
- offers problem resolution suggestions that help you keep to the scope of the EHR project

Project governance

Because an EHR system is highly complex and touches so many individuals in the healthcare organization, project governance is both essential and natural. Project governance refers to the individuals involved in the implementation, those who have ultimate authority for changing the course of the project if necessary, those who ensure user input and champion adoption of the process, and the individuals who are responsible for managing the details.

Involvement

Project governance must reflect all stakeholders and their needs. By their nature, EHR systems are focused on clinical information, the lifeblood of a healthcare organization. Clinical information either drives or relies upon most other information available in healthcare organizations. Clinicians should be the primary stakeholders in EHR implementation. But health information management professionals, patient financial services representatives, compliance officers, and many others play critical roles as well. For example, if the EHR cannot produce an accurate representation of the "health record" to respond to a subpoena or court order, the organization could be in serious trouble. If financial auditors, compliance managers, registrars, or others cannot navigate through the record to find specific information or trace the flow of information in time, many indirect care functions and other functions critical to the viability of the organization will suffer.

Your organization can engage different stakeholders in a variety of ways in the EHR project. One way is to identify all stakeholder categories and then seek out representatives from each category to be "resource" persons. In some cases, you may ask them to participate in or appoint them to a formal committee to provide direction or input. However, you can tap others to offer specific expertise in infrastructure preparation and process improvement/system build. You can ask others to respond to certain issues; test out screens, reports, processes, and training materials as they are developed; or even just offer support and encouragement to others. A "just-in-time" approach is a good way to think of using the variety of stakeholders as resources.

Authority

Although many people need to be involved in the EHR project, you need someone who has the ultimate authority for the project, as well as a formal chain of command. Although executive management has ultimate authority with respect to any system, organizations typically have an executive sponsor for a project of the scope of an EHR. This individual is the conduit between those performing hands-on implementation and the executive management group. The executive sponsor should be actively engaged, but preferably not the key stakeholder for the specific component of the EHR or the steering committee chairperson. The executive sponsor needs to be a neutral party—someone who can build bridges and resolve issues at the highest level. For example, if you are implementing a patient care system for nursing care and documentation, you don't want the chief nursing officer to serve as the executive sponsor.

User input

The executive sponsor cannot and should not be expected to have day-to-day operational responsibility for the EHR project. Unlike other information system implementations, however, the organization may want to share the day-to-day operational responsibility or matrix responsibility among a few individuals (two or more). Frequently, an EHR implementation will have a steering committee, a full-time project manager, and possibly a project management staff.

The steering committee is the primary source of user input. A clinician often chairs the formal committee. The role of the steering committee generally is to make specific decisions relating to how users use the system. The success of a steering committee, however, is to have clear expectations about what decisions it can make and what kinds of decisions it can delegate to the project manager or other staff. Steering committees may also work through specific task forces/ad hoc use of representative stakeholders as resource persons. For example, there may be a task force that works on nursing care screens, another one that works on reporting requirements, and another that represents physician interests in access and documentation. You'll also need to have teams develop interfaces, design the database, run cable, and install devices, but these groups represent the technical aspects rather than the clinical user requirements. The steering committee's main responsibility is ensuring that the implementation meets functional requirements.

Responsibility

A project manager is an individual responsible for keeping the project on track: on time, within budget, to scope, and for specified functionality. This person needs to have strong leadership and change management skills. The project manager needs to work hand-in-hand with the steering committee chairperson and executive sponsor.

The EHR project manager relies upon many other individuals, both those who work within the facility and those who work outside the organization. Internal resources include user representatives, stakeholder resource persons, the chief technology officer (CTO), and informatics leads (the medical informatics professional or medical director of information systems, the nursing informatics professional, and any health informatics professionals within the organization). External resources include EHR vendor representatives, other contractors, and potentially regulators, union representatives, auditors, and others.

Project manager

Executing the tasks required for implementing an EHR is the job of the project manager. This individual is appointed to this role and must have the skills to manage a large project and an appropriate reporting relationship within the structure of the organization.

Sources for the project manager

The EHR project manager may be a professional that is assigned one project after the next within the organization. If this is the case, you must understand the full scope of the project and the required amount of time to manage it. EHR projects can take from several months to, more typically, several years to implement. A project manager assigned to the EHR project generally cannot be working on other projects and cannot be expected to assume a new project any time soon after appointment.

Alternatively, because EHR systems require so much time to carry out and have significant ongoing maintenance activities, you may want to recruit internal or external candidates as a project manager specifically to oversee the EHR project. Project managers primarily must be able to fill the roles of facilitator, leader, coach, manager, accountant, systems analyst, team builder, and communicator. As with the professional project manager, the person recruited for the EHR project manager position must have full-time responsibility and commensurate authority. This is not the job for a department manager or supervisor to take on in his or her "spare time." The project manager must devote full attention to the EHR project.

Yet another approach to project management is to hire a consultant to perform the major project management responsibilities for a defined period of time. If you outsource project management in this way, however, make sure your contract allows all aspects of the project be turned over to the organization upon completion of the project. You'll also want to ensure that specific individuals receive training in managing the project throughout the rest of its life cycle. In addition, there must still be a specific individual in the organization who has the ultimate authority and responsibility for decision-making with respect to the project. Finally, the outsourced project manager must work full-time on the specific project. Unless the individual is highly skilled and your project is very small, or you are only seeking niche expertise or advice, the consultant's time cannot be divided among many different projects.

Project manager skills

For an EHR project manager, the following five skill areas are most important:

- Leadership. Although management is primarily concerned with consistently producing key results, leadership involves establishing direction and aligning, motivating, and inspiring people. Whether designated the chairperson of the steering committee or given some other explicit leadership role, the project manager is always a leader.

- Communication. This refers to the ability to successfully exchange information verbally and in writing and the ability to engage the listener in understanding and carrying out the message conveyed in the communication. EHR project managers must have skills in all forms of communication because there are so many different participants in an EHR implementation.

- Negotiation. This is important to any project because, by its nature, a project introduces change that you must convince others to adopt. Negotiation is particularly important in an EHR project because of the great variety of stakeholders, who necessarily will have competing interests. Many aspects of a project are the subjects of negotiation, including scope, cost, schedule, changes, contract terms and conditions, assignments, and use of resources.

- Problem solving. This entails both problem definition and problem resolution. A skilled project manager must be able to differentiate between the symptoms and the root cause of a problem. Project managers also must be equally comfortable whether the problem is technical, functional, managerial, or interpersonal. Problem resolution requires identification of potential options for resolution and decision-making concerning the best option. The project manager does not have to resolve the problem alone but usually is held responsible for the ultimate decision, even if that means escalating the decision-making to the executive sponsor. The project manager also is not necessarily the individual who carries out the solution. Very often, the project manager assigns responsibility to someone with specific expertise and then monitors progress to ensure resolution.

- Influencing. The project manager is frequently the only person who has the full scope of the project in mind. As a result, the project manager is often in the best position to anticipate the best course of action for a given situation. Politically, however, the project manager may not have the authority to make the ultimate decision and therefore must use the power of persuasion to influence behavior at least toward consensus on an issue.

Project management processes

Project management is the application of knowledge, skills, tools, and techniques to project activities to meet project requirements. Projects typically have a life cycle that involves the accomplishment of specific tasks.

For the EHR project, this life cycle typically includes the following processes:

- **Initiating processes:** These processes authorize the start of each phase of the project. In some organizations, this is a highly formalized process requiring executive sponsor sign off. In other cases, it is a less formal but still important part of careful project design.

- **Planning processes:** These processes define the specifics of how the project will be carried out. They include understanding expectations for the project outcomes and selecting the best courses of action to attain EHR benefits. Planning involves project timelines, resources, team building, and change management.

- **Executing processes:** These processes are all the tasks that result in achievement of the EHR. This is where the project manager spends most of his or her time, and therefore, it's important to appoint the person before the initiating and planning processes because it is difficult to "pick up" where someone else has left off or to start a project without proper planning.

- **Controlling processes:** These processes ensure that the project is on track. These processes entail monitoring, measuring progress, identifying variances, correcting course, and maintaining documentation concerning issues and their resolution.

- **Closing processes:** These processes formalize acceptance of the project phase or project and bring an orderly end to the phase or project. Closing processes for the EHR should include benefits realization studies, celebration, lessons learned, and, potentially, identification of new projects to be initiated.

Although these processes are listed sequentially and generally follow in sequence, they are not exclusively performed in sequence. In fact, the classic "system development life cycle" (SDLC) is typically described as a cascading series of steps or a waterfall because the process involves investigation of initial requirements through analysis, design, implementation, testing, installation, training, deployment, and maintenance. However, such a waterfall model doesn't work in reality, especially when building systems for knowledge workers, such as EHRs for clinicians because the waterfall model assumes that all requirements can be specified in advance. In reality, however, requirements grow and change through the process and beyond, calling for considerable feedback and iterative review.

Both the project life cycle and SDLC are now recognized as potentially taking several different forms:

- **A fountain model** recognizes that although some activities have to precede others, such as developing the overall design before installing software, there is considerable overlap of activities. Still, many aspects of the sequential model are retained in this approach and may be suitable for smaller EHR projects, such as in physician practices or a nursing facility.

- **A spiral model** emphasizes the need to go back and reiterate earlier stages a number of times as the project progresses. This might be thought of as a series of short waterfall cycles, each producing an early part of the project. As more and more processes are accomplished, the closer organizations become to achieving completion of the entire project. Although this might appear somewhat chaotic, it is much more reflective of the evolution of knowledge-based technology. A project manager must be able to cope in such an environment and, while not reverting back to a waterfall model, ensuring that there is control to the chaos so the project ultimately does get accomplished. This is probably the most common model of EHR implementation today.

- **A build and fix model** includes little planning. The organization develops and implements pieces and parts and then adjusts the items to fit the new design. Such an open-ended project strategy can be risky, but many health information systems implemented to date actually are the product of such an overall strategy. However, this is not a strategy recommended for an EHR.

- **Rapid prototyping** is another model in which the vendor creates a prototype that looks and acts like the desired product in order to test its usefulness. Once the prototype is fully refined, it is discarded and the "real" product is created and implemented. This is generally not a strategy for implementing an EHR system, although if the organization agrees to serving as a beta site, the vendor may perform some aspects of rapid prototyping.

- **An incremental model** is one in which the organization discusses the final model, but it creates and tests sections of the project separately from each other. This approach is good for finding errors in user requirements quickly, since the organization solicits user feedback for each state of the project. It is not uncommon for an EHR to be implemented in phases so that the project reflects some of this approach.

In many cases, organizations may deploy some aspects of more than one of these strategies in an EHR implementation that is especially large and complex.

Team building

Although it's important to have the right person for the job of project manager, your organization also wants the right people on the team or teams to support the project manager and do much of the actual execution. For an EHR project, there are several considerations relative to team building, including identifying needed teams, selecting the right people, facilitating the team, dealing with conflict, and achieving success.

Identifying the needed teams

Because an EHR captures data from multiple sources and supplies information used at the point of care and to support decision-making, teams must consider virtually everyone who is involved in care giving. As previously noted, not every user group needs to be involved in every team or attend team meeting. You may use representatives of various departments and specialties as resource persons when needed. However, you do need to identify core teams. These generally include, at a minimum, a physician advisory team, a nursing documentation and quality team, an ancillary service team that can assist in addressing issues with respect to integrating feeder systems, and a support team composed of downstream users such as health information management professionals, patient financial services, risk management, quality assurance, and compliance—to name a few.

Selecting the right people for the teams

When identifying people to serve on the teams, consider the following:

- Can the individuals be team players?
  Although the project manager will lead many of the teams, one person can't oversee all teams at all times. Many teams will need to have leaders who can also facilitate discussion and action items, so consider which individuals possess leadership skills when you appoint team members.

- Do the individuals support EHR?
  Individuals who support EHR and can commit the time to the project make good team members. However, some organizations ask a curmudgeon to join the team because if the organization can convince that individual of the benefits of EHR, the individual may help convince other skeptical staff members. Such a situation is particularly true for clinicians, and even truer for potential physician users. Members of the medical staff know their colleagues well. If those on the fence see a curmudgeon convinced of the importance and benefits of an EHR, many more will be comfortable following suit.

- Do the individual's characteristics blend well with others so the team will produce results?

- The organization needs an appropriate complement of personal characteristics that will blend well and produce results. Figure 3.1 illustrates the breakdown of a team by the dominant personal characteristic of each of its members. Ideally, every team needs at least one of each type, or projects will never get off the ground, never finish, or never accomplish specific tasks. Finally, you must involve appropriate subdisciplines and supporting cast members. Although not every team necessarily needs a member of the IT department, for example, these individuals from IT do need to be actively engaged in the planning process to understand and appreciate what is required.

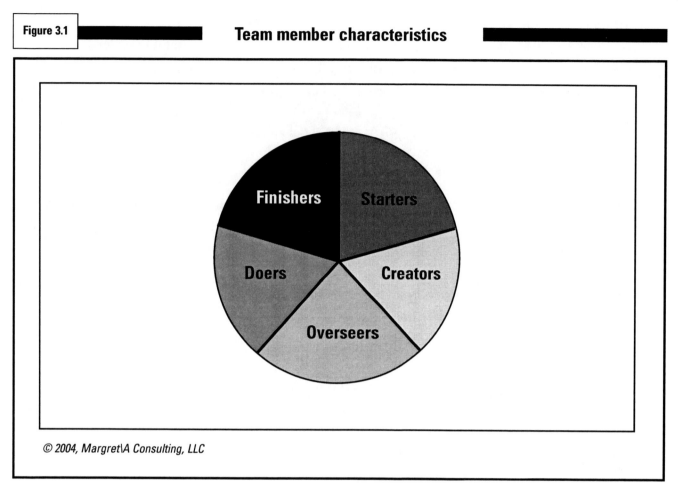

Figure 3.1 · **Team member characteristics**

© 2004, Margret\A Consulting, LLC

Facilitating the teams

Facilitation is an important aspect of the role of both a project manager and the leaders of individual teams. In fact, facilitation training may be an effective precursor to starting up the teams. Effective facilitators are flexible, adaptive, proactive, responsive, and resilient. They establish structure for the team, set the pace of task completion, help team members interact with one another and with other teams, keep the focus, are concerned about individuals as well as the overall focus, and help provide direction and validation for the work being performed.

Dealing with conflict within teams or across teams

Dealing with conflict is an important role for the team leader/facilitator. Organizations need to realize that conflict is inevitable and, in many cases, healthy, as it helps raise issues that it might not otherwise address.

Conflict can be constructive when individuals raise important issues and work together to find solutions. Constructive conflict can also draw out people who may otherwise be indifferent to an issue. In some instances, conflict can actually help build cooperation as people learn more about each other.

However, conflict is destructive when it takes attention away from the primary activity of the team, undermines morale, reduces cooperation, or leads to irresponsible and harmful behavior. Most experts suggest that leaders can resolve or avoid conflict if they meet it head on; that is, they recognize that conflict exists, set goals surrounding the issue of conflict, agree to disagree if necessary, use the conflict to promote creativity, discuss differences openly, stress the importance of following policy, obtain more information where needed, and, ultimately, turn the conflict into a positive experience.

Achieving success in teams

We construct teams because one person or group cannot address all aspects of the EHR implementation alone. Much of the advice provided so far is to help teams achieve success. Some other issues that are often problematical include the following:

- **Holding effective meetings.** It seems as if healthcare organizations cannot survive without meetings. People often start to hate them and attend only grudgingly, an attitude that rarely leads to success. Most organizations could avoid meetings today if people were willing to keep themselves up to date by reviewing project status on their own, but time often forestalls such activity. One way to help overcome this issue is to construct well-designed minutes that are easy to read and to the point. Minutes should reflect actions and only describe discussion where there is a significant opposing view. Send details associated with the actions to the specific person or group charged with carrying them out. Focus meetings on identifying issues and solving remaining problems, not providing information people should have read on their own. Strict adherence to this policy will get across the message that people need to come prepared to meetings or not come at all. If no one comes, the project managers will make decisions. This may sound harsh, but members will get used to this approach and appreciate it.

- **Establishing goals.** Everyone has his or her own agenda and brings that agenda to any team. In fact, without these different agendas, there would be no need for a team. But the end goal must always be kept in sight. One good way to ensure that different agendas ultimately contribute to the common goals is to establish these goals up front with the team through consensus, then continuously refer to them throughout the remaining team activities.

- **Accepting consensus.** It will be impossible to achieve complete agreement among every member of every team. But if team members understand up front that the process must achieve consensus and that agreement will be the deciding factor for moving forward, most tasks can result in consensus. A project manager or team leader/facilitator needs to recognize when the group achieves consensus. It will not be a unanimous vote, but rather by the realization that everyone is basically saying the same thing, although possibly in a different manner.

Figure 3.2

A word about virtual teams

Figure 3.2

Because healthcare organizations must operate on a 24x7 basis and are often composed of several different facilities, the virtual team has become an important ingredient to add to the mix of team building. Although there is nothing like shaking hands with people or providing a big bear hug, meeting in person for every activity is both impossible and unnecessary. There is much technology that can support virtual teams, including audio-visual equipment for meetings as well as groupware to share documents. Virtual teams may actually be more motivated to get the job done because of the desire for connectivity with others.

Virtual team leadership, however, must not forego some of the important elements of on-site teams. Communication becomes very critical. Coaching, support, recognition, and celebration are imperative but often neglected by new virtual team leaders. It may be that these activities are actually put on task lists for the team leaders to remember to do. Virtual team members must also always have the ability to determine project status. Virtual also does not mean unimportant, an excuse to delay, or to avoid assuming responsibility for tasks accepted. It is important to establish a code of conduct for all members of the team, whether on site or virtual. Treat each member equally.

Project planning

Much of the discussion so far in this chapter has centered on engaging people to perform the necessary tasks for implementing the EHR. But organizations must establish an overall plan of approach and then a detailed plan. For a project of the size, scope, and complexity of an EHR, formal project planning methodology is a must. Document the project plan and keep it up-to-date at all times. Whether you use formal project planning software, use a word processing table, or construct a spreadsheet, the project plan must be able to support the various aspects of ensuring task completion on time and within budget.

Overall plan of approach
An overall plan of approach will include identifying expectations and targets, planning phases and general timeframes, estimating the overall level of effort, and agreeing upon a conversion strategy.

Step one: Identify expectations and targets

Some planners refer to this step as a work breakdown structure (WBS), where you must identify all distinct project deliverables necessary to meet the project scope. The EHR vendor contract will likely describe these, at least at a high level. You must understand these expectations and targets in order to meet your contractual obligations or you risk penalties in the form of cost overruns and other problems.

Expectations and targets may include end-state factors, such as how the organization will phase in an EHR, how many new users will it train and by what date, and how many physicians need to use the system in order for the healthcare organization to accept the system is finally and successfully implemented. Expectations and targets, however, also include technical aspects, such as the deadline for installation of the network infrastructure, the deadline for customized templates, external knowledge sources to set up appropriate interfaces, or with whom and how the organization will share data externally to set up trading partner agreements and potentially business associate agreements. The project manager should collect all such expectations and targets—both from the vendor and from the user community.

Step two: Establish phasing and timeframes

Ultimately, each task will have specific dates and possibly even times associated with them for completion. Overall, however, you must establish phases and overall timeframes. Although the project life cycle is not necessarily sequential, it is very important to identify the major phases and how they may, in fact, cycle or spiral throughout the duration of the project.

Phases differ from project life cycle processes in that the processes repeat for each phase. A phase in an EHR project is more typically associated with those aspects that entail a specific set of related tasks.

An example of phases for infrastructure preparation would include upgrading the network, buying and installing servers, and making necessary modifications to the physical plant.

You'll also need to make workflow redesign and process changes. One phase associated with this may be to identify opportunities for improvement. A second phase may be to evaluate what solutions the planned EHR offers for various workflows and process. A third phase may be to identify specific aspects of the EHR that the vendor must customize to meet the organization's specific requirements. Another phase, potentially performed in conjunction with the third, is to write policies and procedures for how users will make changes in their workflows and process in order to most effectively use the EHR. Time each of these phases to be in concert and ready for subsequent phases of the project.

"System build" encompasses many tasks that organizations can group into phases. Different teams will simultaneously perform many of these tasks.

In many cases, you'll want to perform testing, installation, training, and pre-live conversion activities in phases as well. In some cases, you may need to install a piece of the system in a test environment, train a subset of users, and then thoroughly test the piece of the system. In other cases, it may be possible to complete a portion of system build, test it, and then install in final form and provide training.

Establishing overall phases and timeframes helps keep everything from happening at once or nothing happening at all.

Step three: Estimate the level of effort

Once you clearly identify expectations and targets and place them into overall phases and time-frames, you must estimate the level of effort needed to achieve them. Again, the EHR vendor that has considerable implementation experience can provide good insights for this. However, your organization should consider your own experience with major projects and make adjustments where needed. For example, if the vendor indicates that it will take two people one week to review and modify the data dictionary, but your experience with similar projects is much longer or shorter, you should plan your level of effort accordingly. You may need to add people to the task or extend the duration of the task.

Be cautious, however, when you deviate too much from what the vendor suggests. Unless you have considerable experience with very similar projects or the vendor has minimal experience with your type of organization, it may become problematic if you speed up, slow down, load up, or shrink resources. Attempting to accelerate a project beyond what the vendor can truly support will lead to disappointment. Alternatively, slowing down the project too much causes loss of momentum and often user dissatisfaction.

Step four: Establish conversion and turnover strategies

During the overall planning for the project, identify conversion and turnover strategies.

Conversion refers to how users will gain access to previous health records or health information. The patient population, level of interest in research, and technical aspects that dictate cost help determine which approach is best. Strategies include the following:

- Support historical paper record retrieval until no longer requested by clinicians. Your organization will expect that staff will use paper records only for reference and that they will record new information in the EHR. This conversion strategy is simple to execute and tempting to use because it appears to be the lowest cost method. However, it requires the continuation of a paper-based record system potentially for a very long time, reducing the probability of gaining cost savings through staff reduction or other productivity improvements. In addition, it is risky because those individuals who resist using the EHR could actually be documenting in the paper charts without the organization fully realizing that they are doing so.

- Backload paper records by

  - Requiring clinicians to abstract and record needed information into the EHR. This may seem like an impossible strategy, but many organizations have used it successfully. Because clinicians know their patients and know what information they need, they can be judicious about what information they abstract. In an extreme example, a clinic marked each record once the clinician had seen the patient after EHR "go-live," and would not pull the record again except by special request. This was a strong incentive for the clinicians to perform their abstracting.

  - Using abstractors to load specified information into the EHR. This can be effective because it minimizes the risk that clinicians won't abstract the information. It is also a very costly process and one that carries some risk that the abstractor may make errors or that a standard set of data to be abstracted is insufficient for a given patient. Although the paper records should be readily available for a period of time, clinicians may rely on the fact that the abstraction process is complete and accurate and may miss information as a result.

  - Scanning specifically identified documents into the EHR. It is generally less costly than the abstraction process and yet still provides a baseline set of information to be available for first time use of the EHR. The primary drawback is that if the EHR truly contains a set of structured data, the scanned documents do not contribute well to later processing of that data for clinical decision support systems (CDSS).

Another factor is to plan how much to backload. Patient activity should be the primary determinant—and may vary by specialty. For chronically ill patients, it may be necessary to backload a full year or more of data. For more acute types of cases, it may be possible to backload only the last episode of care.

You must plan for the retention and storage of paper records as well. Unless the entire record is scanned into the EHR, in which case you could destroy the paper records, you must make plans to determine how and where you will keep the original record. Once the records become inactive, you must retain them for the period of time the organization has established as its retention period, or at least to comply with the statute of limitations. Warehousing, microfilming, or mass scanning may be options.

- Maintain a dual record system until patients become inactive. In this strategy, paper records for all continuing patients are maintained until the patient is no longer active, but the EHR is used for all new patients. Although this is similar to supporting historical paper record retrieval, it acknowledges use of the paper records. In general, this system is not very satisfactory in gaining clinician adoption of the EHR. There may be some clinicians who have very few new patients on a regular basis and will find it difficult to keep up with how to use the system, especially as the organization adds new features over time.

The above strategies address the transition from paper records to electronic records. An organization might also have data in electronic form that needs to be converted to the new EHR. In this case, you may need to convert the data itself. Determine what data is in electronic form, whether you can convert all data to the EHR, or whether the data can be accessible in another way. If you must convert data, there are special data conversion companies that can perform the process for you, and the EHR vendor may have recommendations as well.

Turnover strategy is related to conversion but somewhat different. Turnover refers to how and when new users will start using the EHR. Turnover strategies include pilots, phases, straight turnover, and pathways.

Many organizations discuss using a pilot strategy. The term "pilot" can mean different things to different people. If this equates to an "early phase in," then the turnover strategy involves implementing the complete system for a small number of users, such as one office or even one physician, one department, one nursing unit, etc. Carefully select which place will be the site of your first phase. For example, the organization may solicit volunteer clinicians, volunteer units, or departments or may make decisions based upon expressed or implied need. However, if it is truly the intent of the organization to "test" through a pilot and potentially pull the plug, then this is a true pilot, and can be a dangerous strategy. It is also one most vendors will not support. Because a true test requires at least 90% of the system to be built, few vendors are willing to go to this much effort for the possibility that the organization will not conduct the rest of the project. Likewise, the organization will have spent considerable resources for little gain.

Straight turnover is another strategy, in which everyone implements the EHR at the same time. For a small facility, this may make the most sense. Larger facilities, however, may find it a difficult strategy to manage. Furthermore, implementing in phases allows lessons to be learned in the first phase that contribute to smoother implementations in subsequent phases.

Another turnover strategy is phasing in a pathway through functionality. Clinical messaging may be the first phase, document imaging the second, CPOE a third, etc. This is essentially the migration path previously discussed. These pathways may also be phased in or implemented in straight turnover—the choice often determined by the complexity of the phase.

Create a detailed plan

Once you've determined the overall approach to the project, identify the detailed tasks. Expectations and targets mean results. Tasks are actions. They have a deadline date, but no duration or time, associated with them. Tasks, however, do have duration of time over which the task is performed.

Project planning tools

There are many ways to construct project plans. You can use a variety of software to support project planning. Microsoft Project® is a widely used program and one that is quite sophisticated, but word processing tables or spreadsheets can also be used. There are also other vendors who sell project-planning software. Some integrate with Microsoft products, including Project® and some with Outlook®, so that team members can post their own progress and manage their own set of tasks. Some project planning software includes other groupware tools, and some are Web-based. Most project-planning software is based on the classic Gantt Chart, which is illustrated in Figure 3.3. Many also have a variety of views for the project manager, including new "dashboard" types of views, which allow the viewing of multiple aspects of the project status, as illustrated in Figure 3.4. However the plan is constructed, there are two primary sources of plan data and usually several components to the plan.

Sources of plan data

One source of plan data is the EHR vendor. As noted in the description of expectations and targets, the vendor contract should specify, at least on a broad scale, what the deliverables are. Most organizations take these broad targets and deliverables and elaborate upon them so they become specific targets or milestones.

Gantt chart illustration

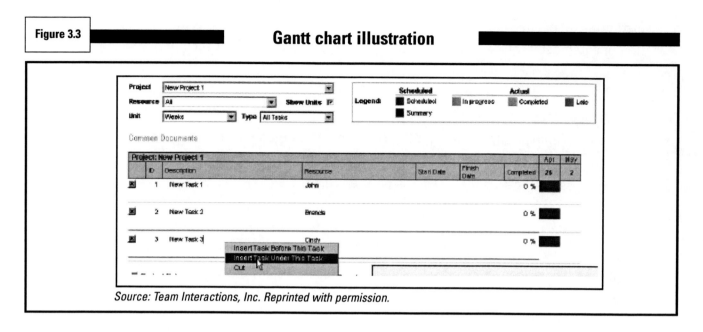

Source: Team Interactions, Inc. Reprinted with permission.

Dashboard example

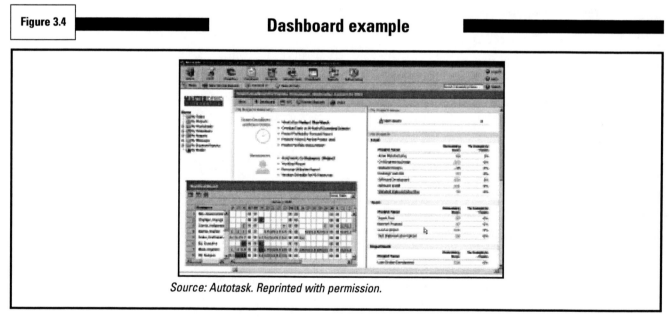

Source: Autotask. Reprinted with permission.

Vendors may also supply a detailed project plan—and offer to manage it for you. While the vendor's detailed plan can be helpful, you need to make the plan your own and manage it yourself. The vendor will manage its components of the plan, but overall, you must manage your own activities and those of the vendor.

The second source of plan data, then, is your own organization's experience. Although few organizations implement an EHR twice, most organizations carrying out an EHR have experience at least with instituting other large projects. These might not even be technology projects, but building construction or enterprise acquisition. Whatever they are, the project plans for such projects can help at least with the process of detailed planning, if not the exact steps.

Plan components

The project plan typically has at least five components. Sometimes the project plan is also used to track issues, in which case the plan is extended by additional components. Most organizations prefer to keep an issues log separately and this book discusses them separately.

The main project plan components include, in order, as you would identify them:

- Milestones—These are the targets or deliverables that contribute to the overall accomplishment of the EHR project. Milestones are associated with a deadline date. Identify them on the project plan first so that you can establish tasks to accomplish each milestone. Milestones are relatively stable throughout the duration of the entire project.

- Tasks—These are the actions to achieve each of the milestones. Tasks will have a start and end date and often will have a tracking component that matches progress against the expected duration. Plan tasks as thoroughly as possible, but realize that you will need to add tasks as the project progresses. A key task for the project manager, however, is to ensure that added tasks are not beyond the scope of the project. Generally, tasks added after the initial planning reflect subtasks or more detail associated with performing a major task. Sometimes organizations must add tasks because of unexpected events. Project managers typically designate these as added tasks to determine whether they contributed to cost or time overruns or they were due to other factors.

- Dependencies—these are often plotted on a project plan, especially those that are automated. A dependency is a relationship between two tasks that shows that one task must be completed before another can begin.

- Resources—these are typically assigned to each task. Resources may be as simple as assigning an individual to perform a task, or as complex as hiring a contractor. One issue you must address when identifying resources is whether you'll pinpoint one individual or a team as primarily responsible for performing a task. If you develop project plans as part of the EHR steering committee's responsibilities, it is very common for the members of the committee to want to populate the "resource" section of a plan with all the various people who may be involved on the team or as resources to the team. There is often a tendency to not want to assume responsibility. It's best to identify a single individual as responsible for each task, even if tasks need to be split into subtasks where each member of a team has assigned responsibilities. A one-task/one-resource approach makes it easier to track the cost of the resources and to monitor progress. One person needs to be accountable for a task, even if that person is a team leader or a lead staff member to a group of employees. Some project plan software allows for detailing the cost of each resource and tracking actual time spent (thus cost of resources). Each organization needs to decide whether this level of detail is necessary.

- Budget—in addition to the level of resources planned and actually used, you must plan other budget elements. Some project managers use the project plan to track all budget elements, others use separate budgets. A budget is critical, and benchmarking against the budget is important whether you track resource utilization and direct costs or only direct costs. Despite the enormity of the EHR project costs, some organizations plan a budget and then do not track actual expenditures. Once again, this is up to the organization, but some controls on actual v. planned expenditures seem prudent. Part of the problem is that the EHR project may truly be a migration path where it is not always clear what part or parts comprise the EHR. Over time, the parts can become muddied and exact expenditures not clear.

Progress reporting and issue tracking

In keeping with the purpose of the controlling phase of project management, the detailed project plan is used to monitor project progress and track issues. Most project planning tools have a Gantt Chart component that tracks progress against task duration, as illustrated in Figure 3.3. Some of these tools will even convert this into a PERT (Program Evaluation and Review Technique)/CPM (Critical Path Method) chart that will help you assess the impact of a change in task completion on the overall completion of the project. The idea behind PERT/CPM is that there are certain tasks that are critical and other tasks that are subsidiary. Any change in the critical tasks impact the ability to get the project done on time/on budget. Subsidiary tasks do not have such an impact. This helps a project manager prioritize the monitoring activity. Subsidiary tasks provide some slack in the overall project completion. Of course, if these tasks go so far over time or budget, they too can become critical impediments.

There are two important components to progress reporting and issue tracking. One is the progress monitoring and reporting and the second is issue identification and resolution.

Progress monitoring and reporting

Monitoring project progress requires the cooperation of all persons assigned to perform tasks related to the EHR project. However, a project manager cannot rely solely on self-reporting of progress. People get busy and may forget to report, or they may over- or under-estimate their progress depending on their personal perspective. A significant part of the project manager's role is not only to track actual progress, but to coach, find additional support if necessary, and recognize efforts—all of which need a personal touch, whether by e-mail, phone, or in person (and usually some combination of all three).

Progress monitoring also means progress reporting. An online project management tool allows everyone to see project progress in real time. However, the EHR steering committee and executive sponsor will probably want a summary of progress on a regular basis. This summary should hit the high points, identifying where progress is lacking as well as where significant progress has been made. It is a good idea to have standard report form so that people receiving it do not need to spend a lot of time reading it to get the essence of what they want to know. The progress report also serves as the basis for the meeting agenda—not the actual reporting (which was discussed above as inappropriate use of meeting time) but rather how to manage where progress is in trouble and to celebrate achievements.

Issue identification and resolution

Identify lack of progress or insufficient progress (including associated cost issues) on one or more tasks as an issue. There are also many other types of issues that will arise. Issues may be that an interface does not work properly or that there is suddenly a new upgrade to third-party software that no one was anticipating. Issues can be large or small, but you need to track them until they are resolved.

The project manager should track issues and be responsible for seeing that they are resolved. The project manager should also know when to bring issues to the EHR steering committee, executive sponsor, or others.

For both project progress and issue tracking, the EHR vendor doing the implementation may offer to physically manage the documentation. Although vendors should have their own project plans and issue lists that they track, the healthcare organization implementing an EHR must manage their own project plans and issues. Although it is certainly not the intent of the vendor to claim resolution of an issue that is not fully resolved or more progress than actual, each party has a perspective. The project manager needs to retain the healthcare organization's perspective and reconcile differences with the vendor.

Project scope

In conclusion, project governance and management are all about ensuring that the EHR is accomplished as intended. This means that it performs the functions intended, achieves its expected benefits, and does so within the timeframe and budget approved or as modified.

Once you've established project governance and management and laid out the detailed project plan, it is time to begin the actual project roll out.

CHAPTER 4

Infrastructure Preparedness

CHAPTER 4

Infrastructure Preparedness

After establishing a governance and project management structure, preparing the hardware and network infrastructure to accommodate the EHR is typically one of the first steps in the actual implementation. In conjunction with building maintenance and construction/physical plant personnel/contractors, IT staff primarily perform this task. However, the design and implementation of the hardware and network infrastructure must conform to the needs of the clinical users. Users' concerns include selecting the right human-computer interfaces, placing wireless access points appropriately, making it convenient to get to a printer, providing virtually instantaneous response time for the network, and ensuring availability of new and old information. The EHR project manager works with IT and users to ensure that the infrastructure supports their demands. In some respects, this part of the project calls for the project manager to become a translator between two foreign languages. Highly technical IT "lingo" and clinical needs are almost as different as any two foreign languages.

Infrastructure preparation includes acquisition and installation of necessary hardware. Because an EHR is designed to eliminate the paper record and all associated processes as well as enhance functionality, your objective is to upgrade the network infrastructure to achieve high reliability and instantaneous response time. You'll need to plan for and carry out any physical plant changes needed to accommodate new equipment. Infrastructure preparedness also includes software delivery preparation such as writing any interfaces necessary to share data with feeder systems. As a participant in this process, this chapter helps you

- plan and implement effective hardware architecture
- identify and address issues with respect to network upgrades
- recognize when it is necessary to make physical plant changes to accommodate new hardware
- build necessary interfaces using interoperability standards
- take delivery of and prepare to install software

Hardware architecture

Infrastructure preparation involves planning and implementing the required technical environment to operate the EHR system. This preparation includes decisions about the overall architecture, storage management, network configuration, physical plant (including data center) upgrades, and human-computer interfaces.

Overall architecture

Applications vendors will normally specify the hardware on which their software operates most effectively. Typically, this includes specifications for

- database, network, and other servers
- storage
- network configuration
- client workstations and mobile, portable, and wireless devices

Vendors will typically specify specific brands or compatibility with certain operating systems for database, network, and other servers. For example, if the vendor uses an Oracle database, it can run on virtually any platform but may perform best on a Sun or Hewlett-Packard server. Vendors may also describe optimal storage processes, including size of memory, online disk space, and other forms of offline and archival storage. An EHR vendor should also work with you to ensure that the network is configured properly. For a small physician office, an EHR may run well on a network with a simple hub and spoke design, but a larger office or small hospital may need switches or routers. An integrated delivery system will require a comprehensive network that is meticulously planned, implemented, and maintained. Vendor products also determine the type of clients that a client/server can use. For example, some EHR applications will not run well on a thin client. Personal digital assistants (PDA) are good examples in which either Win CE or Palm O/S, but not both, is specified.

Be aware of vendor recommendations when planning the overall hardware architecture. Within that construct, however, there are important considerations that only the healthcare organization can make.

For example, one fundamental decision is whether to create a new hardware design from the ground up, to supplement the current legacy hardware, or to develop a transition plan to achieve the required infrastructure. Although you may decide during the planning stage of EHR design and selection to replace, upgrade, or transition the infrastructure, you may have to rethink this if the EHR acquisition process lasts an extended period of time. Some EHR selections can take 12–18 months or even several years. If this is the case, revisit the hardware design at the point of infrastructure preparation.

Figure 4.1 provides a checklist of considerations for replacing, upgrading, or transitioning the legacy systems.

| Figure 4.1 | Hardware architecture considerations |

Consideration	Yes	No
1. Does current equipment meet minimum EHR vendor specifications for capacity, performance, etc.?	Potential for use in transition	High probability of less than positive results
2. Do limitations in the legacy system* impact the ability to use and achieve value from newer systems?	Candidate for replacement	Candidate for replacement
3. Could you convert the legacy mainframe system to a server on the network for back office functions?	Potential for use in transition	Candidate for upgrade
4. Are there sufficient staff resources available who know the legacy hardware?	Potential for use in transition	Candidate for replacement
5. Can you open legacy systems through Web-based portal technology for a transitional period?	Potential for use in transition	Candidate for upgrade
6. Is the manufacturer of the equipment still in business/expected to be in business for a reasonable period of time into the future? (Is the hardware a brand name?)	Potential for use in transition	High probability of problems
7. Are there software solutions (e.g., middleware) to overcome legacy hardware issues?	Potential for use in transition	Candidate for upgrade
8. As cost of hardware goes down and approaches commodity status is the cost of maintaining the legacy system greater?	Candidate for replacement	Candidate for upgrade
9. Is the legacy hardware still under warranty?	Potential for use in transition	Candidate for upgrade
10. Is the migration path for the EHR applications in synch with the migration path for hardware? In other words, is replacement more of an eventuality than an immediate necessity?	Retain until software requirements drive hardware change	Candidate for upgrade

© 2004, Margret\A Consulting, LLC

*Legacy system:

A system that is based on older hardware and software designs and equipment. This may be a mainframe system with terminals.

Some suggest the definition of legacy system is one that works. It introduces yet another change that EHR implementers must manage for full adoption of the EHR.

Although the name of the game typically is to make the most of the information technology you have, implementing an EHR can be a different scenario. The EHR is a mission-critical system like no other. Often, direct caregivers who have never used a computer system before must use the system. In addition to requiring that they learn how to use new equipment, the EHR system will create many changes in the caregivers' workflow and processes. These processes are critical to patients' lives—and support staff need to understand this factor.

Although it's a monumental task to create an EHR system with totally new hardware architecture, doing so will allow you to build a scalable infrastructure that you can modularly extend to meet future needs as the EHR expands. Integrating a new design into the existing infrastructure, no matter how well done, can be risky as the EHR expands in its use and size and as the technology changes. Attempting to manage with older devices can also be a bigger and more costly project over time. In fact, a good way to evaluate the need to replace, upgrade, or transition is to evaluate the initial cost of the hardware and the total cost of ownership (TCO). Figure 4.2 identifies factors in TCO of hardware, especially as it relates to EHR systems.

Figure 4.2   **Total cost of hardware ownership**

Cost factors	Upgrade	Replace
1. Initial acquisition cost	Cost to upgrade	Cost to replace
2. Supplies (e.g., paper, ink, tapes)	# devices multiplied by cost	# devices multiplied by cost
3. Service options	Maintenance cost	Maintenance cost
4. Support cost	# FTE/service calls	# FTE/service calls
5. Associated storage costs (e.g., cost of housing equipment/resultant output)	Cost of storage space	Cost of storage space
6. Associated work space costs (e.g., footprint on nursing unit, carts, travel time to access)	Cost of work space	Cost of work space
7. Ongoing customization costs as new applications are added	Customization costs	Customization costs
8. Cost impact on other systems	Cost impact	Cost impact
TCO		

© 2004, Margret\A Consulting, LLC

Part of the cost of retrofitting an infrastructure is that it usually never quite meets the standards of newer systems in terms of reliability and performance. Because the EHR is used for direct patient care, it is must be as reliable as instantaneously having a blank piece of paper on which to write. Users expect that EHRs will process data at the speed of brain synapses. A system that is perceptively slower than pen and paper or the clinician's thought processes will fail to engage users. This will lead to less than satisfactory adoption and, as a result, less than intended benefits.

Proprietary v. open systems

Another important consideration in the overall EHR architecture is whether hardware and software components are based on proprietary or open solutions. Once again, the organization either made this decision earlier in the process or realized that it would address it early in the infrastructure preparation.

Some EHRs are designed specifically to function best in a proprietary environment. In this case, a single vendor designs component applications that work together seamlessly. If you introduce a non-proprietary component, it may require a vendor to write an interface that may never be fully satisfactory. Use of proprietary solutions often leads to a roadblock in system upgrades, maintenance issues, and potentially a short or limited system life. If the vendor of proprietary applications does not have an application you want, the choice becomes one of either struggling with an interface or waiting a long time for the vendor to develop the application. If you introduce another application, you must maintain it with each upgrade performed on the original platform. As the mix becomes broader, it will become more difficult to maintain various interfaces.

"Open systems" may refer either to those based on an industry-recognized standard or to literally open source architecture. Systems based on industry-recognized standards, such as Windows, are compatible with a variety of software applications designed to the standard. Open source means that the source code in which the software is written is accessible and otherwise complies with the criteria of the Open Source Initiative (OSI).[1]

Don't confuse Open Systems Interconnection (OSI) with the Integrating the Healthcare Enterprise (IHE) initiative. Figure 4.3 describes these concepts.

| Figure 4.3 ▮ | **Open systems interconnection v. integrating the healthcare enterprise** ▮ |

Open Systems Interconnection (OSI) reference model, developed by the International Standards Organization (ISO),[2] refers to the ability of computers to communicate over local and remote networks. The model defines seven layers in its framework:

7—Application layer supporting end-user processes

6—Presentation layer provides independence from differences in data representation

5—Session layer manages connections between applications

4—Transport layer provides transparent transfer of data between hosts

3—Network layer provides switching and routing

2—Data link layer encodes and decodes data packets for transmission

1—Physical layer conveys the bit stream, or electrical, light, or radio signals, through the network hardware

At one time, most vendors agreed to support OSI, but it was too loosely defined and proprietary standards were too entrenched. Except for the OSI-compliant X.400 and X.500 e-mail and directory standards, which are widely used, the standard now serves as a model for other protocols.

Integrating the Healthcare Enterprise (IHE) initiative has grown out of the fact that although vendors supplying EHRs and their components write to standards for interoperability (e.g., Health Level Seven [HL7] and Digital Imaging and Communications in Medicine [DICOM]), vendors can implement those standards in any manner that is most compatible with their technology and architecture. The results are standards-compliant systems with incompatible architectures. Integrating these components still requires costly and time consuming adjustments.

In 1998, the Healthcare Information and Management Systems Society (HIMSS) and the Radiological Society of North America (RSNA) collaborated in a joint initiative now called IHE to define how the HL7 and DICOM standards will be implemented. The IHE Technical Framework defines the tasks that must be accomplished for various integration profiles (e.g., scheduled workflow, patient information reconciliation, consistent presentation of images).[3]

Price/performance considerations

Another factor in the overall architectural design is that of price/performance equipment purchasing. Any organization should ensure that it gets the best price for what it purchases. However, the lowest price does not always mean a good deal. Performance includes proven and tested technology with support to back it up. Price/performance compromises can end up being more costly in the long run.

In reviewing the vendor specifications for the infrastructure, always make sure that the equipment purchased at least matches, if not exceeds, the minimum performance requirements as specified by the EHR vendor. For example, if the vendor indicates that the EHR will not perform well on thin clients, plan to buy clients that at least have the minimum processing and storage capacity indicated by the vendor.

Device re-use and disposal

Some healthcare organizations looking at a major overhaul of their hardware infrastructure will face managing obsolete equipment and potentially redeploying equipment.

If your plans call for donating equipment or selling it to employees or others, be sure you have fully eradicated any protected health information (PHI) that may be on a hard drive. Reformatting the hard drive is insufficient for this purpose. In fact, many healthcare organizations remove the hard drive and either store it or physically destroy it before donating the rest of the device. Hard drives are not that difficult to remove and not that costly to replace.

In redeploying equipment around the organization, it may be acceptable to simply reformat the hard drive, especially if new users will have similar access privileges. This may be the time, however, to upgrade the hard drive.

Storage planning

A major part of infrastructure preparation is preparing for data storage. This includes decisions about storage capacity, redundancy, methodology, management, and location.

Capacity planning

Capacity planning refers to the amount of storage you will need over time for the EHR. Although the EHR vendor can assist you with estimating your future storage needs, there are several important factors to tell the vendor so that it can recommend the right configuration. The amount of storage a healthcare organization needs escalates tremendously when implementing an EHR. There are several contributing factors:

- First, the purpose of the EHR is to collect data from multiple sources and integrate that data. By its very nature, then, the EHR is an application requiring significant storage. It is a good idea to outline all existing feeder systems and their current storage needs. Current storage for most community hospitals without considering picture archiving and communication systems (PACS) and other new clinical applications is between one and three terabytes (TB) per year.

- Second, the EHR is either composed of or connects with many other clinical applications that generate large volumes of data to be stored. For example, storage of images for PACS is huge. And even if the initial implementation of the EHR does include such systems, by definition these systems will eventually be acquired and need to be integrated. Your list of storage needs should include an outline of future information technology plans and expected growth of the organization. It is not uncommon for a community hospital to expect its storage needs to grow up to five TB per year with the addition of these other applications.

- A third consideration is that the EHR is mission-critical. It must supply data to users instantaneously. This means that the EHR must store a significant amount of data online for real-time access. It is generally recommended that organizations plan for three to 24 months worth of online storage capacity. The online storage requirement also means you have comprehensive c ontingency plans.

- Finally, most healthcare organizations hope that the EHR will lead to a paperless environment. Such an environment also requires large-capacity, fully-redundant storage for a long period of time. Many healthcare organizations have not made decisions about how long they will keep their electronic data. Because mass storage of electronic data takes up so much less space than paper files, this has not yet been an issue for most organizations. However, consider two critical elements:

  - First, the longer electronic data is stored, the more likely the medium on which it is stored will deteriorate and cause data integrity problems. It is important to test continuously for the ability to retrieve data and, potentially to have a rotation plan to ensure durability of the media.
  - Second, the more data accumulated, the more difficult it may be to actually process it if needed for other than archival retrieval purposes. For example, if a healthcare organization wants to use 20 years worth of clinical data for a research study, how easy will it be to mine the data that is stored in long-term storage? Although you can keep electronic data for longer than the statute of limitations or medical staff bylaws require, it may not actually be necessary to do so.

Redundancy

A fundamental factor in EHR online data storage is redundancy—of both data and systems to manage the data. Downtime is not tolerable in an EHR environment. Disk arrays, sometimes referred to as "spinning disks," are becoming popular for this purpose. Redundant Array of Independent (or Inexpensive) Disks (RAID) storage is essentially a set of computers optimized to be single-purpose storage appliances that employ two or more disk drives in combination for fault tolerance and performance. There are number of different RAID levels, and their descriptions often vary by vendor. Figure 4.4 offers a description of RAID levels.

Figure 4.4	RAID levels

Level 0—Striped disk array without fault tolerance: Provides data striping (spreading out blocks of each file across multiple disk drives) but no redundancy. This improves performance but does not deliver fault tolerance. If one drive fails, then all data in the array is lost.

Level 1—Mirroring and duplexing: Provides disk mirror. Level 1 provides twice the read transaction rate of single disks and the same write transaction rate as single disks.

Level 2—Error-correcting coding: Not a typical implementation and rarely used, Level 2 stripes data at the bit level rather than the block level.

Level 3—Bit-interleaved parity: Provides byte-level striping with a dedicated parity disk. Level 3, which cannot service simultaneous multiple requests, also is rarely used.

Level 4—Dedicated parity drive: A commonly used implementation of RAID, Level 4 provides block-level striping (like Level 0) with a parity disk. If a data disk fails, the parity data is used to create a replacement disk. A disadvantage to Level 4 is that the parity disk can create write bottlenecks.

Level 5—Block interleaved distributed parity: Provides data striping at the byte level and also stripe error correction information. This results in excellent performance and good fault tolerance. Level 5 is one of the most popular implementations of RAID.

Level 6— Independent data disks with double parity: Provides block-level striping with parity data distributed across all disks.

Level 0+1—A mirror of stripes: Not one of the original RAID levels, two RAID 0 stripes are created, and a RAID 1 mirror is created over them. Used for both replicating and sharing data among disks.

Level 10—A stripe of mirrors: Not one of the original RAID levels, multiple RAID 1 mirrors are created, and a RAID 0 stripe is created over these.

Level 7: A trademark of Storage Computer Corporation that adds caching to Levels 3 or 4.

RAID S: EMC Corporation's proprietary striped parity RAID system used in its Symmetrix storage systems.

Source: Webopedia: RAID, July 28, 2004. Copyright 2004 Jupitermedia Corporation
All Rights Reserved, www.webopedia.com/TERM/R/RAID.html. *Reprinted with permission.*

Storage methodology

Longer-term storage has typically included magnetic or optical media. Magnetic tapes and disks are the oldest form of such storage. Optical disks in various formats have for the most part replaced magnetic media. These optical storage formats include compact disks (CD) and digital versatile disks or digital video disks (DVD). DVDs are a type of optical disk technology similar to the CD but commonly used as a medium for digital representation of movies and other multimedia presentations that combine sound with graphics.

The media can be configured as network attached storage (NAS), storage area network (SAN), content addressable storage (CAS), or a combination of these.

- NAS is a networking architecture that attaches disk arrays to computers. A NAS is economical because it relies on older, well-established technologies, such as the hard drive standard ATA (advanced technology attachment) and Internet Protocol (IP) data networking. It is important to note that implementing a NAS will change your server acquisition strategy and save significant budget dollars due to the minimal amount of storage required at the server level. Increased recoverability via a NAS could also be one of the most significant advantages of this strategy. For example, in the event of a primary server failure, you now have the ability to automatically remount a data set to a hot secondary server. You can measure downtime in this scenario in minutes instead of hours. You can achieve this same result with replication and clustering, but the cost of supporting duplicate hardware and software is much higher and increases the load on the network.

- SAN is similar in concept to a NAS, but it uses newer and faster communications technology, known as fiber channel, to create communications bandwidths of 1 or 2 GB. With a SAN, you can interconnect storage resources across wider physical distances into a shared pool and still maintain split-second response times for end users. A SAN works in a way that makes all storage devices available to all servers on a local area network (LAN) or wide area network (WAN). As more storage devices are added to a SAN, they too will be accessible from any server in the larger network. The server acts as a pathway between the end user and the stored data. Because stored data does not reside directly on any of a network's servers, server power is used for processing the applications, and network capacity is released to the end user.

- CAS is an object-oriented system for storing data that users don't intend to change once stored. CAS assigns a unique identifying logical address to the data record when it is stored. The address is neither duplicated nor changed in order to ensure that the record always contains the exact same data as originally stored.

Storage management

In addition to the storage hardware and how it is configured, you can also purchase software to efficiently manage the stored data. Storage management software provides a view of storage resources from a central console so that storage managers can find and offload data from nearly full to less-full disks—a process typically performed manually. Storage management software is still in it infancy and is expensive. Some estimate that the cost of storage management software is equivalent to 80% of the total cost of the storage itself.

Storage management should also ensure that systems meet industry standards. These standards affect how text, images, and communications pipelines that connect storage components connect to the EHR. Figure 4.5 describes evolving storage standards.

Figure 4.5	Evolving storage standards[4]

Standard	Description
Digital Imaging and Communications in Medicine (DICOM)	This standard enables different computing platforms to share image data. The standard supports conversion of images to digital form and should be sought in all picture archiving and communications systems (PACS), other medical devices that produce images, and document imaging systems.
Serial ATA (SATA)	This is a standard for disk drives that increase their data shuttle rate to 150 Mbps initially, with the potential for speeds up to 600 Mbps. This standard could make tape drives for storage totally obsolete, replacing them with by far faster disks.
Bluefin	This is a vendor-neutral application programming interface that can be used between SANs from different vendors. The standard also increases the reliability and security of storage devices to make them easier to manage.
Internet Small Computer System Interface (iSCSI)	This boosts data transfer speeds among interconnected storage devices and computer running on traditional Ethernet networks. The standard may permit continued use of an existing Ethernet network instead of having to replace it with expensive fiber.

Storage location

Long-term storage, sometimes called legal, disaster recovery, or archival storage, is often placed at a site away from the main facility. Many healthcare organizations store backups off site, but it is also possible to outsource all storage management to a storage service provider (SSP). An SSP is much like an application service provider (ASP) that provides outsourcing of the storage function. It can be a cost-effective means to handle long-term storage.

Network configuration

An EHR implementation almost always triggers a formal network assessment and frequently results in a network upgrade. EHR systems result in many users simultaneously accessing data and performing processes on the data. As a result, you usually need to expand network resources.

Key network performance factors

In general, there are five performance factors relating to networks. These are the metrics upon which you should base your network assessment and justify network upgrades needed for EHR systems[5]:

- Bandwidth is the rate at which information is transmitted through a network, measured in kilobits (Kbps) or megabits (Mbps) per second. This is a property of the transmission medium (e.g., fiber optics, coaxial cable, telephone wire, radio waves), the network topology, and the switching or routing devices used to guide traffic through the network. EHRs demand a greater amount of bandwidth than other applications because they are required to transfer large amounts of data quickly.

- Latency is the time required to transmit data across the network. On the Internet, the number of packets each message contains frequently determines latency. Latency is influenced by the speed of the switches and routers in the network and the physical distance across which the transactions must be sent. Real-time, interactive applications such as EHRs demand low latency so that users can interact with each other easily. Within an LAN or WAN, latency is often referred to as response time.

- Availability refers to the ability of the network to continuously provide passage of data. You can measure availability in terms of the percentage of the time the network is operational or by the average time between failures. A number of factors can render a network unavailable. These include physical damage to the network links or nodes, hardware or software failures, operator error, software errors, and deliberate malicious attacks against the system. You can take steps to harden systems against these failures and develop procedures for restoring network services in the event of failures.

- Security is the ability of a network to provide confidentiality, data integrity, and availability. Availability is described above. Confidentiality refers to the protection of the privacy of data. Data integrity refers to the fact that data have not been altered. Both of these factors are of critical importance in an EHR system. Technical mechanisms exist to address confidentiality and integrity, including authentication, encryption, and access controls.

- Ubiquity refers to the relative accessibility of a network. For an EHR to be successfully adopted, access to the network must be easy for all potential users. Ease of use includes access to human-computer interface devices and a design of the application that makes it intuitive to use.

Network characteristics

Within healthcare organizations, there may be one or more types of networks, each requiring the above key performance factors. Assessing network capabilities for the EHR address whether the network characteristics are the most useful in supplying the performance factors.

Local area network

An LAN is a computer network that spans a relatively small area, such as a single building or group of buildings. When LANs are connected to one another, they form WANs. LANs connect all devices that compose the computer system, including workstations and other clients to servers and other computer devices. LANs are differentiated by the following characteristics:

- Topology is the arrangement of devices on the network. From the most simplistic perspective, these might include a straight line or a ring. There are variations on each of these. Each topology has advantages and disadvantages.

- Protocols are the rules and encoding specifications for sending data through the network. The protocols determine whether the network is "peer-to-peer" or "client/server." Peer-to-peer networks use workstations that conduct their own processing and save their own data. The network allows transmission of the data from one workstation to another. Most network configurations today are client/server, where servers provide the processing and storage to their client workstations.

- Media are used to provide the actual connection between devices that transmit information. Hardwire networks use various cables, such as twisted-pair wire, coaxial, or fiber optic. Wireless networks use radio waves.

Ethernet LAN architecture is the primary type of network found in healthcare organizations. Ethernet networks use a bus or star topology and typically have supported data transfer rates of 10 Mbps. A newer version of Ethernet, called 100Base-T (or Fast Ethernet), supports data transfer rates of 100 Mbps. The newest versions of Ethernet, Gigabit Ethernet, supports data rates of 1,000 megabits per second, or one Gigabit per second (Gbps) or greater. The Institute of Electrical and Electronics Engineers (IEEE) is a standards organization that develops standards in many technical areas ranging from computer engineering to biomedical technology and telecommunications. IEEE has established the standard (IEEE 802.3) for Ethernet designations. Figure 4.6 describes the differences in Ethernet designations.

Figure 4.6   **Ethernet designations**

10Base-2	10 MBps baseband Ethernet over coaxial cable with a maximum distance of 185 meters. Also referred to as *Thin Ethernet* or *Thinnet* or *Thinwire*.
10Base-5	10 Mbps baseband Ethernet over coaxial cable with a maximum distance of 500 meters. Also referred to as *Thick Ethernet* or *Thicknet* or *Thickwire*.
10Base-36	10 Mbps baseband Ethernet over multi-channel coaxial cable with a maximum distance of 3,600 meters.
10Base-F	10 Mbps baseband Ethernet over optical fiber.
10Base-FB	10 Mbps baseband Ethernet over two multi-mode optical fibers using a synchronous active hub.
10Base-FL	10 Mbps baseband Ethernet over two optical fibers and can include an optional asynchronous hub.
10Base-FP	10 Mbps baseband Ethernet over two optical fibers using a passive hub to connect communication devices.
10Base-T	10 Mbps baseband Ethernet over twisted pair cables with a maximum length of 100 meters.
10Broad-36	10 Mbps baseband Ethernet over three channels of a cable television system with a maximum cable length of 3,600 meters.
10Gigabit Ethernet	Ethernet at 10 billion bits per second over optical fiber. Multimode fiber supports distances up to 300 meters; single mode fiber supports distances up to 40 kilometers.
100Base-FX	100 Mbps baseband Ethernet over two multimode optical fibers.
100Base-T	100 Mbps baseband Ethernet over twisted pair cable.
100Base-T2	100 Mbps baseband Ethernet over two pairs of Category 3 or higher unshielded twisted pair cable.
100Base-T4	100 Mbps baseband Ethernet over four pairs of Category 3 or higher unshielded twisted pair cable.
100Base-TX	100 Mbps baseband Ethernet over two pairs of shielded twisted pair or Category 4 twisted pair cable.
100Base-X	A generic name for 100 Mbps Ethernet systems.
100Base-CX	1000 Mbps baseband Ethernet over two pairs of 150 shielded twisted pair cable.
1000Base-LX	1000 Mbps baseband Ethernet over two multimode or single-mode optical fibers using longware laser optics.
1000Base-SX	1000 Mbps baseband Ethernet over two multimode optical fibers using shortwave laser optics.
1000Base-T	1000 Mbps baseband Ethernet over four pairs of Category 5 unshielded twisted pair cable.
1000Base-X	A generic name for 1000 Mbps Ethernet systems.

When assessing network performance, you must consider all the components that make up the network, as each could affect the network's performance. This starts at the cable in the wall connecting all of the workstations and extends to the network closets and network backbone connecting to the equipment in the data center. Support for high-performance networks calls for installation of multimode fiber in the risers that link the data center to the wiring closets. The current standard for wire to the jack in the wall is Category 6 or CAT6. Outdated buildings and bad wiring practices due to a lack of standards, installation by multiple vendors, and constant moving of staff and departments, which is very typical in hospitals, can make this part of the infrastructure preparation a real nightmare that must receive a high degree of attention.

A decision as to the size of the connection to certain workstations is another factor in network performance. For example, retrieving medical images would require 100 MB connections to the workstation, while normal administrative/clerical users might require only 10 MB.

Remote networking

A technical strategy for remote users of the EHR is another element of the overall infrastructure preparation. The success of an EHR depends just as much, if not more, on users who access the system remotely as those within the hospital structure. Data retrieval that takes a long time is more frustrating than it is valuable.

To determine your options, contact your local telecommunications provider because capabilities and recommended configurations can differ depending on location. In addition to advice, they can provide design and implementation assistance. The current trend is that T1 connections that might have been adequate in the past are being replaced with Gigabit speed connections operating over a metropolitan area network (MAN) infrastructure.

Metropolitan area network

As with your LAN, the MAN linking all of your sites should provide mega-bandwidth communication that is highly reliable and redundant. Redundancy is also important in network capability. In this case, redundancy is further enhanced by dual entry into the data center. With an EHR, the objective is to maintain a MAN that is robust enough to support the movement of images virtually anywhere, any time. A MAN can also give you the capability to dramatically improve your data back-up and recovery process by mirroring and storing data off-site. Transporting data to an identical SAN at a remote location provides for an online system back-up available immediately in the event of an outage at the main data center.

Virtual private network

Another technical strategy for remote communications that is gaining popularity is establishing a virtual private network (VPN). A VPN uses encryption and other security mechanisms to construct a virtual tunnel through the Internet through which only authorized users can transmit data in a secure manner.

Traditional remote access methods have proved to be inadequate solutions due to poor performance and support. And, with the advent of HIPAA, data security is a major concern. Today, a VPN is a logical choice for providing remote access to clinical users like physicians at home or in their offices. A VPN offers two distinct technology advantages. First, a VPN uses an industry standard security protocol (Secure Socket Layer [SSL]) to secure electronic transactions. This is the same technology that supports millions of secure online transactions every day in the financial industry. It establishes an Internet infrastructure to ensure confidentiality and encryption of patient information.

The second advantage is that the method of this secure access is available through the use of the common Web browser. This is of particular importance to the end user who does not need to learn a new method of presentation and navigation to access the EHR. In addition, it also eases the set-up and support requirements. Overall, a VPN that leverages existing Internet technology provides a cost-effective and secure solution to providing an electronic health information highway for remote clinical providers.

Wireless area networks

An extension of the hard wired network is a wireless infrastructure, or wireless area network (WAN). This needs to be planned concurrently as part of an overall strategy to provide system access to the EHR at the point of care. Because healthcare professionals are mobile, going to the patient—whether in a hospital bed or examining room—most healthcare organizations are adopting portable devices for users. To make them easiest to use, the portable devices are generally wireless.

It is imperative to design a wireless infrastructure in much the same way that a traditional network infrastructure is designed. Your planning effort should result in a blueprint for the entire enterprise. Even if you decide to start small and implement a WAN in only one department or one area of the facility, it is a good idea to understand the full scope of what an enterprise WAN might look like. You will be surprised at how readily they are adopted and demanded as the standard for all parts of the organization.

Because full coverage of your facility is essential, placing your access points is a major concern in the design. You cannot create a wireless zone, or place other restrictions on use of the network. You can't lose data because of a lost signal, and users won't tolerate brownouts that significantly slow the network down. Hire an expert to perform a detailed site survey and spectrum analysis as the surrounding environment needs to be completely assessed for obstacles that will affect wireless performance. For example, large metal food carts have been known to cut off wireless access. In addition, you must consider electromagnetic interference. Wireless devices and networks can potentially interfere with monitoring devices and other medical equipment.

Several wireless standards have emerged, as summarized in Figure 4.7. The IEEE 802.11 family of standards is most typically used for wireless networks, although Bluetooth may be an important adjunct for certain types of medical equipment. The IEEE 802.11 family of standards provides you with important options.

Consider whether the wireless product is "Wi-Fi certified." Wireless fidelity (Wi-Fi) refers to any type of 802.11 network. When Wi-Fi Certified by the Wi-Fi Alliance, the products are interoperable with each other. Formerly, the term "Wi-Fi" was reserved to describe the 802.11b standard, in the same manner that "Ethernet" is used in place of the IEEE 802.3 standard. The Wi-Fi Alliance expanded the generic use of the term in an attempt to stop confusing people about wireless interoperability.

Remember the potential for interference with monitoring and medical devices. Some experts are concerned about the newer broad (2.4 gigahertz [GHz]) spectrum used by 802.11b and 802.11g. Although these standards push data transmission rates to 54 Mbps, the broad spectrum has greater potential for radio frequency (RF) interference. The 802.11a standard also provides high transmission speeds—up to 54 Mbps—but within the five gigahertz range, which is farther away from the spectrum used by monitoring and medical devices.

Security is also an important issue for wireless networks. The Wired Equivalent Privacy (WEP) protocol was designed to provide the same level of security as that of a wired LAN by encrypting data over radio waves. WEP is available in 40-bit or 128 bit encryption. WEP is not as secure, however, as it was intended to be. It regulates access to a wireless network based on a computer's hardware-specific MAC address, which is relatively simple to sniff or steal. It was also intended to protect data as it is transmitted from one end point to another. However, WEP is used only at the two lowest layers of the OSI model, so it does not offer full end-to-end security. Wi-Fi Protected Access (WPA) is designed to improve upon the security features of WEP. It improves the data encryption capability through use of a temporal key integrity protocol (TKIP) that scrambles keysand adds an integrity-checking feature to prevent tampering of keys. Generally missing in WEP, WPA also provides user authentication through the extensible authentication protocol (EAP). WPA is an interim standard that will be replaced with the IEEE's 802.11i standard that uses a more complex option for encryption (Advanced Encryption System [AES]).[6]

Infrastructure Preparedness

| Figure 4.7 | Wireless network standards |

Standard	Data rate	Modulation scheme	Security	Advantages/disadvantages
IEEE 802.11	Up to 2 Mbps in the 2.4 GHz band	FHSS or DSSS	WEP & WPA	This has been extended to 802.11b.
IEEE 802.11a (Wi-Fi)	Up to 54 Mbps in the 5 Ghz band	OFDM	WEP & WPA	Eight channels are available. Less potential for RF interference than 802.11b and 802.11g. Supports multi-media voice, video, and large image applications better than 802.11b. Relatively shorter range than 802.11b. Not interoperable with 802.11b.
IEEE 802.11b (Wi-Fi)	Up to 11 Mbps in the GHz band	DSSS with CCK	WEP & WPA	Fourteen channels are available (only 11 of which can be used in U.S. due to FCC regulations and only three are non-overlapping). Requires fewer access points than 802.11a for coverage of large areas. Offers high speed access to data at up to 300 feet from base staion.
IEEE 802.11 (Wi-Fi)	Up to 54 Mbps in the 2.4 GHz band	OFDM above 20 Mbps, DSS with CCK below 20 Mbps	WEP & WPA	Fourteen channels (see 802.11b). May replace 802.11b. Improved security enhancements over 802.11. Compatible with 802.11b.
Bluetooth	Up to 2 Mbps in the 2.4 GHz band	FHSS	PPTP, SSL, or VPN	Does not support TCP/IP or wireless LAN applications well. Best suited for connecting PDAs, cell phones, and PC in short intervals. May work well for wireless medical devices.

Modulation refers to transmission technology to blend data into a carrier signal. Frequency-hopping spread spectrum (FHSS) and Direct-sequence spread spectrum (DSSS) are most common in wireless networks. Complementary Code Keying (CCK) is a complementary function in DSSS technology to encode data. Orthogonal Frequency Division Multiplexing (OFDM) is modulation technique for transmitting large amounts of digital data over a radio wave.

Point-to-Point Tunneling Protocol (PPTP) is a new technology for creating VPNs that enhances security when messages are transmitted from one VPN node to another.

Source: IEEE, Wireless LAN Standards. © 2004 Jupitermedia Corporation. All Rights Reserved, www.webopedia.com/quick_ref/WLANStandards.asp. *Reprinted with permission.*

Electronic Health Records: Strategies for Implementation *89*

Consider the number of devices you will need to determine the optimal location of the access points that will provide the greatest signal strength. With proper planning, cabling from the network closets to these wireless access points becomes a very straightforward task. Completion of the wireless infrastructure will allow portable devices to operate in real time just like any workstation anywhere in the hospital or practice.

Physical plant changes

Achieving the expectation of zero downtime and ubiquitous access to the EHR is also made possible by creating a physical infrastructure plan. Although the primary focus will be the data center, you'll need to consider many other aspects of the physical plant. For example, if there needs to be server closets/wiring closets, you must identify and control them.

Despite the advent of wireless portable devices for user access to the EHR, there will remain issues of where to place the device while examining the patient or administering medication. You must place wireless access points within the physical infrastructure. Not all components of the EHR are amenable to the smaller, portable devices—meaning you must plan location of workstations or flat panel monitors as well.

Data center

If the data center needs considerable remodeling or moving, redesign begins with estimating the total space requirement for all equipment. Size and design of the overall physical structure will also dictate security, fire protection, and raised floor systems if you are expanding, refurbishing or building a new data center.

When you identify the full complement of equipment that needs to be located in the data center, you can calculate the electrical and air conditioning (A/C) loads from manufacturer specifications. Important in all of your load analysis is adequate capacity for future equipment that you will need as your data storage and processing power needs grow. Much of the hardware to serve EHR needs is getting smaller, but generally many more devices are needed. Not only does this mean that you may not reduce space, but you may actually need more space for people to move around the equipment easily for maintenance and repair.

Building into your data center infrastructure a superior level of redundancy will go a long way to ensuring your objective of high EHR availability. Interruption of electrical power to your critical computer equipment is the most common failure that a data center experiences. Electrical failures will occur, so you must prepare for them by identifying the single points of failure and then providing protection to minimize the impact. Standard procedure for a data center facility is an uninterruptible power supply (UPS) to handle short interruptions and an emergency generator to cover electrical failures that are long term. Attach a smaller UPS to switches in network closets to ensure uninterruptible power to each segment of your network. As an additional level of protection, equip all servers and other mission-critical devices with internal dual power back-up and separate power feeds in each.

Planning the data center requirements for the EHR is your first critical step in the EHR project because laying the physical foundation can require a long lead time and major capital expense.

Other physical plant accommodations

Although the data center is clearly the hub of the IT activity for the EHR, there are other physical plant accommodations that you will need to evaluate.

One consideration is whether the data center will, in fact, be centralized. Most organizations find this most convenient, although some organizations—especially those adopting a best of breed approach to application acquisition—may permit location/maintenance of servers in user departments. If this is the case, involve the IT team to ensure that all components of security—not just confidentiality, but data integrity and availability (which includes business continuity and disaster recovery)— are addressed.

An organization may also find it convenient to locate some servers or wiring in closets closer to user locations. Evaluate such closets for their A/C capability. Not only do these closets tend to get very hot, but there is frequently minimal air flow, humidity controls, and other environmental considerations. Such closets should also be the exclusive domain of IT. Do not share the closets as storage locations for the cleaning crew, painters, etc. Cleaning and painting chemicals do not mix with sophisticated information technology.

You'll also need permanent or temporary placement of various devices, including wireless access points and housing for workstations. Although further discussed in the section on human-computer interfaces, housing for the devices used by EHR users to interact with the EHR become very critical. These locations need to afford security from both incidental disclosures and from theft. The locations need to be convenient and also be safe to use. Hospitals are notorious for attempting to suspend workstations from ceilings, placing devices on carts, and temporarily putting devices in places that are precarious at best. Making sure that people do not bump into, trip over, or drop them are important safety and security measures. These may seem like rather esoteric issues, but the key to user adoption of the EHR is to make it easy to use.

An important tool to evaluate placement of human-computer interfaces is the floor plan, which should identify all existing furniture and equipment, location of electrical sources, heating and cooling vents, doors and windows, and other factors that may influence placement of devices. Making changes to the floor plan, however, must be done in concert with users. Any change in floor plan introduces change in workflow, and that must be clinically acceptable.

Human-computer interfaces

The human-computer interface, formerly called user interface or input/output device, has become a critical element in EHR adoption. The interface must make the computer easy to learn, easy to use, and adaptable to a wide range of users in varied environments. One of the most notable trends in computing is the variety of computational devices with which users interact. In addition to workstations and desktop PCs, users are faced with laptops, or notebooks, and a multitude of mobile devices such as PDAs, tablets, and computers on wheels (COWS). Devices can differ greatly, most notably in the sizes and resolutions of displays, but also in the available input devices, the stance of the user (standing or sitting), the physical support of the device (sitting on a desk, mounted on a wall, or held by the user), and the context of the device's use (point of care, at a nursing unit, physician's lounge, or at home/in the office).

Another challenge with so many different devices is maintaining uniform user interface for an application across a range of devices. Uniform interfaces are important for applications to retain a common look and feel regardless of the device on which it is operating so users can quickly learn to use a familiar application on new devices. Usually this is managed by the software vendor who will also list devices that they will support.

Probably the best strategy is to roll out these devices gradually and to stage various pilot situations where users can match the device to the application's use and workflow necessary to accomplish their daily tasks. A lightweight wireless device may be the top priority of one group of users. Another group might require high resolution to view images. Yet other users may identify a long battery life as essential. Nothing is worse than betting on a technology for a specific mobile device and spending many capital dollars only to find the fit is not right. This is not to mention the user frustration that will develop with the EHR implementation and the need for replacements for the devices that lay idle. After you test these devices, develop standards so that there is consistency of the products purchased to maintain an effective support program.

Another consideration is the associated navigational devices, monitors, microphones, biometric devices, etc., that you will need to make the device work. For example, if a user wants to work on a PDA, you may need to supply a keyboard attachment. Consider whether dictators will be working in a quiet radiology reading room or in a busy emergency department when you set up microphones for speech recognition. If you are adopting biometrics, consider whether users will wear gloves most of the time. These are just a few of the considerations that need to be made, especially as human-computer interfaces become point of care technology (POCT).

Software delivery

When the hardware, network, and physical plant infrastructure is nearing a state of readiness, it's time to begin the preparation to accept software delivery. This includes timing issues; preparing development, testing, and training environments; and planning for change control (or configuration management) and integration steps.

Timing

It's important to time the software delivery step to synchronize with other project activities related to the actual EHR software implementation process. Other upcoming project activities will establish how you will need to configure the system databases. But before you can do that, you must establish standards for vocabularies and data comparability measures. These may be driven by the nature of clinical protocols, introduction of clinical decision support, design of structured templates, regulatory and compliance data and information requirements, and many other factors. The EHR project plan, developed in concert with the vendor, lists all these tasks, and you should use it to identify when it is best to take delivery of the software.

Development, testing, and training environments

Most healthcare organizations have learned from experience that any development work, testing, and training should not be done on the production environment. Too many things can go wrong that can impact current processes. Therefore, most organizations either use a separate server or create a separate area on a server for development, testing, and training.

- Development refers to the customization of the software to meet your specific requirements and the writing of interfaces to connect different applications. This may be called "system build" and is addressed fully in Chapter 6.

- Testing is also a crucial step and is often required in the contract for acquiring the EHR. All aspects of testing an EHR are covered in Chapter 7.

- Training is not only a one-time process when the EHR is first implemented: It's an ongoing process not only for new users, but for changes. Training environments include not only the technical environment but also both physical and virtual classrooms. Training strategies are discussed in Chapter 9.

Change control

During the software build or configuration phase and subsequent testing, many changes or patches to the actual software may be made. In addition, the vendor may periodically send new versions of the software. That is why attention to software maintenance is essential upon initial loading of the software. This entire process must be policy driven to ensure that users understand responsibilities and procedures. This includes the establishment of a change log to record and track software changes so you can manage and control them. Communication and scheduling of the actual change is critical both during the implementation and after "go-live." This is especially true in a phased implementation where active development continues on. During the implementation, you must apply program code changes very carefully especially when testing and training takes place. At some point, you must freeze the code to maintain system stability. Continual patching of the system leads to the never-ending process of testing.

As the project draws closer to "go-live," you will need to establish system operations to support the production environment. The final aspect of system implementation is the completion of all system documentation including policies and procedures. This documentation, together with training to ensure proper communication and understanding, serves two purposes. First, you need instruction from a systems operations perspective, and second, help desk staff need to know how to handle any issue that users present. Adequately trained technical staff is critical to user acceptance and satisfaction with the system.

Appendix A at the end of this chapter provides a policy, procedure, and set of forms for managing the change control process.

Integration

Virtually any EHR implementation requires linking with other systems. Even with a core solution, there are always integration issues with other applications that will require the sending and receiving of data to and from the EHR. An evaluation of your strategy for this integration is critical to moving forward in development of the EHR.

The basis for this integration is the work of a key standards organization, HL7, and the use of a middleware tool called an "interface engine." The broad objective of HL7 is to provide comprehensive standards for the electronic exchange of data among healthcare applications. HL7 message-based data integration traditionally has been used to transfer data from one system to another to minimize duplicate entry, maintain data integrity across various systems, and collect transactions for processing. These interfaces are coded and mapped in the "interface engine" to provide the necessary integration. With the introduction of the EHR, you must consider the entire process of real time data integration needs when building the technical infrastructure. The organization must determine which components it will need to manage and control the data transfer process, which at times can be quite complex. This will require HL7 expertise and careful planning to define your specific integration requirements.

Because the EHR will also need to integrate with images, electronic prescribing systems, and potentially other applications, it is also important to recognize the standards typically deployed for interoperability within those domains.

DICOM has already been discussed as the standard for interoperability between imaging systems. It was further mentioned that HL7 and DICOM are working together (under the IHE initiative) to promote seamless interoperability between HL7 messages and images.

Another important standard is the National Council for Prescription Drug Programs (NCPDP) SCRIPT standard for transmitting prescription transactions to retail pharmacies. This is the predominant standard for electronic prescribing systems (and the standard required under the Medicare Prescription Drug, Improvement, and Modernization Act of 2003 [MMA]). Much like HIPAA and its financial and administrative transactions and code sets standards, the MMA requires adoption of standards when electronic prescriptions are used under the Prescription Drug Program, Part D (starting with pilot testing in 2006, with an effective date in 2007, and a compliance date in 2009). Although hospitals will use HL7 to communicate medication orders to the clinical pharmacy within the hospital (whether solely for order communication or for CPOE), physicians will need to use NCPDP SCRIPT to send prescriptions, refill/renewal approvals, and other related transactions to retail pharmacies. This includes both prescriptions written in the physician's practice, and those issued upon discharge of a patient from the hospital or emergency department or from a hospital outpatient facility.

The end result

Attention to the building of the physical infrastructure will require time and careful planning. It is important then to focus on the process of building the infrastructure and using the right technology to meet the established clinical and business objectives. An effective technical infrastructure will also be one that employs standards to avoid interoperability issues and uses versatile networking solutions that can adapt to change without substantial cost. The end result must be an infrastructure that supports the delivery of care where and when it is needed across a range of devices and locations.

End notes

1. Open Source Initiative, The Open Source Definition (*www.opensource.org/docs/definition.php*).

2. International Standards Organization, Open Systems Interconnection (OSI) reference model (ISO 7498-1).

3. P. Vegoda, "Introducing the IHE Concept, *Journal of Healthcare Information Management*, Vol. 16, No. 1, (January 2002), pp. 22–24.

4. A. Joch, Nine Tech Trends: Storage, Health Care Informatics, February 2003.

5. Committee on Enhancing the Internet for Health Applications: Technical Requirements and Implementation Strategies, *Networking Health: Prescriptions for the Internet*. (Washington, DC: National Academy Press, 2000).

6. J. Retterer and B. W. Casto, Practice Brief: "Securing Wireless Technology for Healthcare," *Journal of* AHIMA, Vol. 75, No. 5, May 2004, pp. 56A–56D.

Title: Configuration management		Number:
Originator:	Date Originated:	Approved by:
Date(s) Reviewed:	Date(s) Revised	Distribution:

Summary

A formal change control process ensures both that the security measures of systems will work when they undergo change and that applicable upgrades, patches, and other controls are implemented when they become available. [Name of Provider] uses a formal change request and tracking process to ensure that all changes are addressed in a timely manner and security is an integral part of all system changes.

Policy

I. A formal change control process is used to eliminate/reduce disruptions and maintain acceptable levels of service for normal operations during the implementation of changes in information systems by monitoring and managing the following:

- Frequency of changes
- Length of time required to implement changes
- Impact of changes on business units
- Changes resulting in problems
- Concurrent changes

II. A formal change control process contributes to the effective and efficient management of [name of dept, such as Information Technology Services] resources, including providing

- central inventory of all information systems and their current upgrade status
- central coordination and control of all change management functions
- assurance that change controls meet vendor's contractual obligations
- testing and validation that security features and controls have not been altered or compromised as a result of a hardware or software change

III. A formal change control process provides a central repository for all change data that will be used to measure and report on the effectiveness of the change management system by evaluating

- impact of business unit objectives
- percent of successful changes
- change window overruns
- number of unrecorded changes and percent that failed
- number of required backouts and percent that failed
- number of unplanned/unscheduled outages due to change

Procedure

I. Change management processes consist of seven major elements that begin with completion of a formal Change Request to schedule changes and end with actual change implementation and subsequent review and analysis. A [*identify who, such as Quality Assurance Analyst*] manages the seven major elements of change management:

- Change request
- Technical and business assessment of change
- Management approval of change
- Documentation
- Testing
- Implementation
- Reporting

II. Change requests

- To ensure that adequate lead-time is provided for change implementation, a Change Request must be made to [*who?*] and must be made well in advance of the need for the change. See the Change Categorization and Required Lead Times form appended. Changes must be requested via the [*use as applicable: automated change management system or Information Systems Change Request Form*].
- All change requests will be entered into the change management system.
- All change requests must be accompanied by a technical and business assessment for the change.
- A change window is a block of time set aside to perform hardware and software maintenance, upgrades, etc. To the extent possible, the change window should be employed for patches and minor changes.
- No changes may be communicated directly to the vendor.

III. Technical and business assessment of change

- Technical assessment is the process of evaluating the technical risk, effect, and feasibility of implementing the change at the desired time. This is often determined through meetings conducted by the [*identify who, such as Quality Assurance Analyst*]. Low-level changes may only require a brief discussion between the Change Implementers and the [*identify who, such as Quality Assurance Analyst*]'s discretion as to whether a change warrants an actual meeting.
- Business Assessment is the evaluation of a planned change for the amount of risk and impact the change will have on the organization's customer community when implemented.

IV. Management approval of change

- Only changes requested on a formal change request form and fully documented with a technical and business assessment will be evaluated.
- Designated individuals will evaluate the change request and indicate approval of change as requested, require the change to be delayed, or disapprove the change.

V. Documentation

A. All of the following changes will require not only management approval, but full documentation:

- New computers installed
- New applications installed
- Different configurations implemented
- Patches and updates installed
- New technologies integrated
- Updated policies, procedures, and standards
- New regulations and requirements
- Identified and implemented fixes for network or system problems
- Different network configuration
- New networking devices integrated into the network

B. Documentation of changes will be retained for the life of the applicable hardware or software.

C. Documentation of changes that are delayed or disapproved must also be retained for the life of the hardware or software.

VI. Testing

- All changes must be tested in the test environment prior to moving them to the production environment. Monitoring of the change test is the process of tracking and documenting the final test of the change prior to actual change implementation and communicating the results of the test to all concerned parties.
- All changes must reflect the same or greater level of security enablement as the original system. Testing must include a test of the security features.

VII. Implementing

- All changes will be implemented with the same diligence as the original system.
- Changes must be monitored and tracked.

VIII. Reporting

- The duty to report the results of change implementation are equivalent to the duty to report new system implementation.
- The evaluating the overall operations and achievements of both the change and the entire Change Management System. These achievements are determined through reports created from change records and statistics.

CHAPTER 5

Workflow Redesign and Process Changes

CHAPTER 5

Workflow Redesign
and Process Changes

Unlike any other information system application, the EHR should and will improve the underlying clinical tasks performed by healthcare organizations. In fact, an EHR being sold to "not change how you practice" is unrealistic. Why would anyone spend considerable resources on a product that would not help make any quality or performance improvements? Changes, however, must not negatively impact the quality of care, patient safety, or the patients' and users' satisfaction with the healthcare experience.

This chapter covers workflow redesign and process change, which are not isolated steps. Implementing an EHR is not a sequential process; rather, you must conduct workflow redesign and process changes in lock step with both the infrastructure preparation (covered in Chapter 4) and the system build (covered in Chapter 6). Workflow redesign and process changes identify the necessary infrastructure updates and feed directly into system build. This chapter is designed to help the organization adopt an EHR plan and implement EHR-triggered workflow redesign and process changes. Specifically, the chapter

- describes the importance of quality and performance improvement
- provides tools for effective workflow redesign and process change
- supplies change management techniques
- helps make necessary clinical transformations with adoption of the EHR
- offers suggestions for policies, procedures, and user manual development

Importance of quality and performance improvement

The healthcare industry has had a long, although somewhat checkered, history of quality and performance improvement. Efforts to ensure quality have gone by many names, and organizations have adopted many different tools and techniques over time. Figure 5.1 offers a laundry list of such methodologies.

Figure 5.1

Sampling of quality improvement methodologies

- Balanced scorecard
- Benchmarking
- Best practices
- Business process reengineering
- Continuous quality improvement (CQI)
- Cultural change
- ISO9000
- Knowledge management

- Learning organization
- Management-by-objectives
- Outcome-based evaluation
- Program evaluation
- Quality circles
- Statistical process control
- Strategic planning
- Total quality management (TQM)

Some healthcare organizations follow one methodology very strictly. Others use pieces of several methods as they deem necessary for a particular focus. Small organizations may not use any formal methodology but still conduct quality assurance or performance improvement activities.

Key outcomes

This book is not concerned with the methodology chosen or not chosen, rather, it stresses that you use whatever formalization of effort leads to successful outcomes. The University of Massachusetts Medical Center (UMMC) has developed a facilitator's guide to "clinical process redesign," in which it outlines five outcomes of process redesign efforts in healthcare. These outcomes are very applicable to EHR implementations as well. The following outcomes as described by UMMC have been adopted for EHR implementation[1]:

- Clinical outcomes are the results of treatment interventions. For the EHR, positive clinical outcomes are the primary goal. For example, The Leapfrog Group supports the adoption of CPOE because the system should reduce medication errors and the potential for adverse drug events (ADE). Likewise, the Medicare Prescription Drug, Improvement, and Modernization Act of 2003 (MMA) calls for adoption of electronic prescribing standards to ensure the quality and cost effectiveness of the new Medicare Part D program. And many hospitals have implemented barcode medication administration to improve the likelihood that they will give the right drug to the right patient at the right time in the right dosage with the right frequency.[2] Although medication errors have received considerable attention from the Institute of Medicine's patient safety reports,[3] there are many other clinical outcomes. For example, there is a need to ensure successful surgical interventions, laboratory test optimization, and appropriate differential diagnosis. These outcomes can be aided by information made available through processing in clinical decision support systems (CDSS). In the UMMC schema there are quality of life measures that address physical and social functioning, bodily pain, vitality, and the impact and perceptions of physical and mental health. Many organizations use the SF-36 health status profile developed by The Medical Outcomes Study to measure and benchmark the health status of their patients.[4] EHRs can help organizations remember to monitor the health status of their patients by providing appropriate reminders and alerts. Applying functional outcome indicators directly into the EHR and subsequently redesigning and changing affiliated workflow and processes provides an opportunity for the entire health care delivery system to operate more effectively and efficiently. As a result, you should notice an improvement in clinical outcomes, quality of life, and organizational productivity. Adoption of these processes also can go a long way toward assisting an organization in delivering both efficient and effective health care.

- Patient satisfaction assesses the overall patient experience with the services provided during an episode of care. Many new EHR users express concerns about workstations and other human-computer interface devices getting in the way of or becoming barriers between the caregiver and patient. These issues can be overcome by engaging the patient in the process of documentation. Statistics also point to the fact that patients do not always understand why they must continually repeat information to which they believe caregivers have access. They also are especially interested in having electronic communications with providers.

- Organizational climate is described in the *Clinical Process Redesign* guidebook as how people feel about their work environment and predicts organizational performance. It is a predictor of organization's willingness to change, its readiness to accept an EHR, and its likelihood of realizing positive results/achieving benefits.

- Costs and utilization outcomes are defined by UMMC as the efficient use and provision of patient services during the healthcare process. These are often measured in terms of patient length of stay and variable cost per case. UMMC indicates that the appropriate ordering of tests and services by care providers and the efficient operation of areas providing these tests and services are the key factors contributing to favorable cost and utilization outcomes. With respect to EHR implementation, you could measure cost and utilization and take appropriate corrective actions in order to achieve a positive return on investment (ROI), higher caregiver adoption rates, and increased user satisfaction. Many organizations, in fact, track user adoption to identify problem areas. Many organizations implementing an EHR will also conduct formal surveys of users to determine initial readiness issues and ongoing concerns.

Key components

Another way to describe the impact of the EHR on quality and performance improvement is suggested by Kremsdorf in The Five Rights of Effective Patient Care.[5] Dr. Kremsdorf suggests that "effective patient care is the result of the coordinated efforts of a patient care team, all of whose members have what they need to provide optimal care," and suggests that "there are five key components that are essential for this system to work smoothly." These "five rights of effective patient care," as they relate to the EHR include the following:

- Right clinical data—is necessary for success. Kremsdorf notes that health care has become increasingly data-driven, that some data are more important than other data, and that knowing both on what data to focus and what data to use is critical. An EHR should be able not only to capture data from multiple sources but to process the data in meaningful ways to supply the right information. But EHRs do not, in themselves, produce the right information—they must be programmed to do so, and modified and updated on a continual basis to ensure that new evidence is factored into the data processing. The saying "data rich and information poor" is often used to describe healthcare organizations. A critical factor in designing the workflows and process changes to use an EHR is to capitalize on the available data and convert it into useful information. Merely capturing more data will overwhelm the majority of users and often does not serve any useful purpose.

- Right presentation—involves the right data, delivered at the right time, in the right format, in the right sequence, and in the right context. These are critical components for designing EHR workflows and processes—and factors that must also be flexible. For example, rules must take patient specifics into account and not be intended for the entire patient population. Building a robust CDSS that fires alerts constantly even according to the best founded and most well-intended rules will be ineffective and ultimately the cause of great user dissatisfaction. A CDSS, however, that fires alerts at the right time in the right context is very helpful. The alerts also must be presented in a format that various users can use. Alerts that fire according to rules for medical students and house staff may be designed to require immediate attention. However, you may also want to consider specific rules that provide only informational use as an option when an attending physician is logged into the system. For many healthcare organizations, the process to establish rules and alerts is not thoroughly examined during evaluation of these technologies. The right presentation of alerts based upon pre-determined rules is a dynamic process during which both of these components must be continually evaluated and addressed.[6]

- Right decision—is the main focus for the use of CDSS and the EHR. However, such applications do not and should not make the decisions for the caregiver but instead offer the intelligence for the caregiver to use to make the right decision. Although there is no substitute for human intuition, heuristic thought, and innate intelligence, they can be supplemented with the right data and subsequent information, in the right presentation format in order to provide well-designed decision-making support. It is the task of the healthcare organization to apply these factors in their EHR systems.

- Right work processes—are factors that contribute to correctly implementing the right decisions. These work processes may be requirements for bar coding the delivery and administration of medications, for forced-choice from a pre-established medication or lab test formulary, evidenced-based steps in clinical pathways, or essential and critical questions to ask or observations to make when assessing a patient presenting with chest pain. The right work processes will decrease rework, lower errors, and reduce the number of steps in a process. In its basic form, this is workflow redesign and process change. When data and work processes are integrated into a single, seamless process, you can enhance coordination and cooperation achieve optimal results.

- Right outcomes—are the feedback mechanisms that ensure that the data, presentation, decisions, and processes are, in fact, right. Although it is good practice to track EHR system utilization, mere use does not guarantee the right outcomes. You must measure results against prior results to determine whether the EHR has had a positive influence.

The five outcomes and the five right factors are important, but they do not by themselves achieve or guarantee the results. Rather, results must be planned, sold, implemented, and managed, and the systems must be supported over time.

Planning for workflow redesign and process change

Planning to redesign workflows and to make process changes requires facilitation, teamwork, innovation, integration, and extensive attention to detail.

Facilitation

Facilitation is encouraging users to search and identify the right workflows and processes for use in the EHR system. Chapter 3 describes project governance and planning. Even if the project manager or other individual assumes the task of facilitating workflow redesign and process change, the key role is that of change manager. The facilitator needs to understand the underlying workflows and processes. This does not necessarily mean the facilitator is an integral part of those workflows and processes. In fact, a facilitator who is one of the intended users will very likely bring personal biases to the process of workflow redesign and process change that may not result in considering all alternatives and selecting the best one. Alternatively, if the individual knows nothing about the flow of information throughout health care, it will be very difficult to select the right tools, offer guidance on their use, draw out good ideas, stimulate innovation, and support integration.

Teamwork

Teamwork requires building openness and communication with all individuals involved in the EHR implementation and adoption. Workflow redesign and process change need to be performed in lock step with infrastructure preparedness and system build activities. This is critical for the success of these projects because the specifics of each component part are dependent on each other part. Consider the following simple example: A user group decides to place shelves above every patient's bed for computer devices; as a result, the physical plant must determine the feasibility from an infrastructure and construction standpoint; finally, patient safety is asked to determine whether there is any risk to the patient relative to the positions of the shelf and the bed. Likewise, physician users of CPOE systems need to express the importance of CDSS in order to effectively and efficiently use CPOE systems, or the process of CPOE will appear to be one of physicians taking over a clerical task.

Every clinical area obviously must be involved with respect to its own workflow redesign and process changes. However, you must involve other downstream users of the information. For example, if a nursing documentation system is easy for nurses to use but physicians cannot navigate through it to find critical pieces of data, or if users can't print out the information in response to a subpoena as documentary evidence of work performed, or if an auditor cannot review the documentation for completeness, the system overall will not yield the best possible outcomes. Priorities may be identified, but every use of data must be considered and planned for. As such, all potential users must ultimately "touch" the workflow redesign and process changes that are proposed. Ultimately, you must achieve alignment among interest groups and development of consensus (which is where a strong facilitator can help).

Innovation

Innovation could well be put at the top of this list because an appreciation for taking a critical look at current workflows and processes and literally "thinking out of the box" with respect to how they might work better is the most important factor in achieving the right redesign and changes. Unfortunately, too many healthcare organizations are unwilling to make the necessary workflow redesign and process changes necessary to achieve the optimal benefits from EHRs. Organizations have complained that systems were not designed by caregivers in current practice or have not kept up with today's best practices. Other organizations decide that they are unique, have special needs, and will customize a system so that it looks and operates just like their current, paper-based practices. Although systems may have design flaws and organizations do have special needs, it is important to work with the system as proposed and to find the right balance of practice change and customization. You must never sacrifice quality and patient safety, but recognize the unwillingness to accept change is very often a symptom of resistance to change.

A key step in achieving innovation is to prepare users in advance of acquiring the EHR for upcoming changes. A good method for doing so is to have them review their own workflows and processes, look for redundant, time-consuming, and error-prone tasks, and offer changes as appropriate, irrespective of the technology that may be coming. This allows users to see the issues that exist today without the factor of change influencing them. It also achieves buy-in. *They* made the change—the system didn't! In addition, they can help adapt the system to the new workflows and processes they propose and not revert back to the old way.

Finally, the fear of losing one's job because of computerization is still as prevalent today as it was when computers were first invented and introduced more than 50 years ago. Although computers have primarily added jobs, responsibilities change because of computers, and if an individual is unwilling to make the necessary changes (i.e., learn new skills/acquire new knowledge), then it is possible that the organization may move individuals to another position or that jobs will be lost through attrition. Unfortunately, the notion of staff savings is still very strong in the minds of executive management—fostered by vendors who tout just that. Even more unfortunate is the fact that rarely does the vendor projection match reality. When an EHR vendor suggests that a hospital may be able to reduce nursing staff by 3.75 FTEs, it typically means that among all the nurses, each nurse may be saved a few minutes of time per day in processing paperwork. It is impossible to reduce nursing time by a fraction of nurse. But the reduction does mean that each nurse should be able to spend more time on direct nursing care. It may also mean that you won't need overtime or temporary help. (EHR may help reduce the number of clerical staff who perform solely paper-related functions, such as pulling and filing charts. However, even in these cases, the staff members are often re-deployed and performing other functions, such as document scanning.)

Integration

Integration refers to bringing disparate components together. But not only are these disparate components information systems applications that do not interface with one another, they are also departments or specialties that have traditionally not interfaced, or not interfaced well, with one another. By definition, an EHR is a system that captures data from multiple sources, integrates it, and provides meaningful information to users from that process. The intent of the EHR is to integrate and to overcome the specialization, compartmentalization, and silos of information and work processes. Health care is frequently compartmentalized because the complexity of the human condition has led to specialization. That does not mean, however, that you shouldn't coordinate separate processes. The patient is still a single system of heart, lungs, skeleton, skin, brain, etc. What happens to one organ or subsystem impacts the entire system. Likewise, health care needs to focus on the entire patient with coordinated care. This perspective hopefully should help in removing barriers for team members to work together for the common good, which is the objective of a patient-centric, information-rich EHR system.

Attention to detail

Attention to detail is the final element in planning for workflow redesign and process change. Although very intelligent people have designed computers and created EHRs that perform wondrous functions, computers in themselves are not intelligent—they only do what they are told. You must program them to perform as humans desire them to perform. As such, when presented with an EHR design and the task of matching workflow redesign and process change to the design of other workflows and processes, all decisions must be accurately and completely documented so they contribute to the build of the system in the manner that will best achieve quality and performance improvement.

Whether it is the project manager, workflow redesign and process change facilitator, or a recorder designated for these purposes, it is essential to communicate what changes need to be made with the programmers, systems analysts, and implementation specialists (the systems' build team). Likewise, as users settle on the workflow redesign and process changes they will adopt, they need to incorporate them into policies and procedures that they will apply when the EHR is implemented. This attention to detail, communication, and documentation will also help reinforce the quality and performance improvement initiatives when it comes time for adoption. EHR project success will be measured against the original objectives and intent, and it could well be the impetus for more technical support.

Tools for workflow redesign and process change

Once an appreciation of the need for workflow redesign and process change associated with EHR implementation exists, you must determine the actual redesign and changes. As suggested in the introduction to this chapter, there are many overarching methodologies for quality and performance improvement. There are also many specific tools—some of which are available in automated form, others of which are simply easy to sketch out on paper or to use via generic computer tools. This section will highlight some of the tools users find most helpful in assessing workflow and processes. This section also introduces a process to ensure that quality and performance improvements are achieved through workflow redesign and process changes.

Steps to achieving workflow redesign and process changes

Steps in achieving workflow redesign and process changes include the following:

1. Constructing cohesive teams
2. Orienting team members to concepts of workflow redesign, process changes, and the potential scope of EHR impact
3. Instructing team members on the objectives, timeframe for accomplishment, and use of workflow redesign and process change tools
4. Identifying opportunities for improvement prior to recommending changes
5. Determining the root cause(s) of quality and performance issues
6. Identifying suitable workflow redesign and process changes
7. Documenting changes to submit to the system build team
8. Incorporating changes into policies and procedures
9. Testing new workflows and processes where feasible in advance of the EHR
10. Training others on new workflows and processes
11. Obtaining pre-"go live" benchmark data to use in benefits realization studies
12. Celebrating success of new workflows and processes

Step one: The EHR project manager in conjunction with the steering committee constructs cohesive teams. The organization must understand the full scope of the EHR implementation before it can establish a representative team. If you plan to phase the EHR implementation, you may not need to create teams in certain areas. The organization must give members the authority, responsibility, and time to work on the team.

Steps two and three: Orienting team members to concepts of workflow redesign, process changes, and the potential scope of EHR impact and then instructing them on the objectives, timeframe for accomplishment, and use of workflow redesign and process change tools is often performed by the project manager and/or workflow redesign and process change manager(s). If the organization is lucky enough to have informatics specialists, these individuals will often head up the workflow redesign and process change teams, perform these functions, and facilitate the overall team effort.

You must preserve the principle of integration. A nursing informatics professional should work with nursing, but not at the exclusion of physicians, other clinicians, and downstream users such as health information management, patient financial services, quality improvement/risk management, compliance, and other such professionals. These others do not have to participate in all aspects of the nursing workflow redesign and process change team, but they should be as active as required. At this point, it may not be necessary to have IT staff participate, especially if there are medical, nursing, and health informatics professionals who can make the translation between clinical and health information processes and information technology.

Step four: Identifying opportunities for improvement prior to recommending changes is an important skill that trained informatics professionals or other facilitators can bring to the workflow redesign and process change teams. Many potential EHR users have a tendency to want to jump right in and identify changes (or offer reasons why there cannot be changes) based on the specific functions the EHR system being acquired supports. If there is any "wrong" approach, it is this. There are two main dangers here. The first has been alluded to—that it is a means to disregard, discredit, or otherwise find a way not to make a change that may be needed (i.e., resistance). The second could be worse—that it is found that the underlying workflows and processes are producing the best possible quality and performance outcomes and that change would not be appropriate. Usually this latter condition is not the case, but you should acknowledge that the risk is present.

The best way to ensure that the opportunities for improvement are identified outside the context of the specific EHR functionality is to conduct the assessment early. Sometimes organizations do this during the evaluation of EHR solutions even before making an EHR selection. Others will do it early in the implementation process to ensure an unbiased viewpoint. There must be a balance struck, however, between keeping team members in the dark as to what an EHR can accomplish and what needs to be changed. Although most potential users have had little experience with computer systems in general and need an orientation to stretch their imaginations and to create an innovative environment, potential users may overestimate the powers of the EHR functionality. They may propose changes that are indeed desirable but not feasible, or at least not feasible with the specific EHR being acquired. Of course, you should have done this reconciliation prior to selection—and that is the primary reason for conducting step four prior to selection.

Identifying opportunities for improvement will often require data collection and potentially benchmarking with other reference organizations or against published best practices. For example, if national data indicate that as many as 44,000 to 98,000 people die in hospitals each year as the result of medical errors[6] and there are roughly 4,000 hospitals, then there are between 11 and 25 deaths per hospital on average. You will want to compare this number with your hospital's actual numbers. Clearly, if your numbers are higher, this is definitely an opportunity for improvement. If they are lower, however, you may first want to ensure that they do not creep up by still considering opportunities for improvement and then decide how much lower you could get your numbers with workflow redesign and process changes. Remember, unless your number is 0, there is always room for improvement. The amount of effort to improve, however, could be incrementally greater the lower your numbers are.

Not every opportunity for improvement is as clear-cut as medication errors. (In fact, medication errors may not be as easy to quantify in your organization, as it would appear from the national data. Not all errors are easily identified or get reported.) Most potential users of the EHR system, however, do have a gut feel or intuition about potential opportunities. A critical factor in identifying these, however, may be fear of blame or retribution. It is essential that staff identify opportunities for improvement in an environment where there is no reproach for identifying the opportunity. This will require a considerable degree of trust on the part of the team members, which needs to be built and facilitated throughout the process. Another way to identify potential opportunities for improvement is simply to collect data about the outcomes of the most important processes performed—and question each one, whether it raises a red flag or not. This approach tends to eliminate the potential for blame.

Step five: Determining the root cause(s) of quality and performance issues is the next step. One of the problems with benchmarking is that it only compares your level of performance to someone else or to what a group considers to be a documented best practice. It does not help you identify the underlying processes that determine the level of performance to begin with. Continuing with the medication error results example, attempt to understand the cause of any errors. For example, you may find that you only have 10 identified errors per year. But if you determine that they are all due to one process where national data would suggest that only half all errors are typically attributed to that process, your level of performance suddenly does not look as good as it did when only the total was considered.

Currently, there is no consistent process among healthcare organizations for detecting and reporting medication errors. Because many medication errors cause no harm to patients, they remain undetected and largely unreported. Still, organizations frequently depend on spontaneous voluntary error reports alone to determine a medication error rate, and the variability of determining error rates in this way invalidates the measurement. In fact, a high error rate could suggest either unsafe practices or an organizational culture that promotes error reporting. (In fact, this is why the IOM study results have such a huge range of potential error.)

Figure 5.2 is a diagram that was drawn from an important medication error study[7] that highlights the root cause of errors, not just their volumes. It is this type of diagram (and others—see next section) that can be helpful in determining root causes.

Figure 5.2	Root cause analysis of medication errors

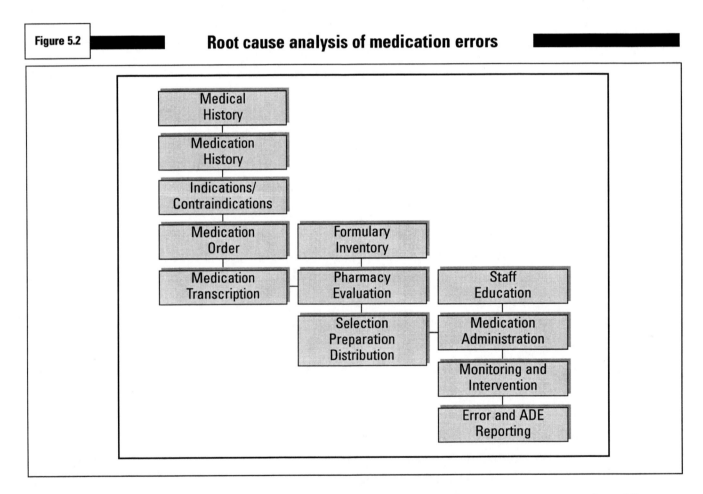

Figure 5.3 is another example of how an organization documented current processes and workflow involved in the process of writing a prescription. Each area that has potential for error is referenced to a narrative description.

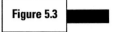 **Example of workflow and process assessment for prescriptions**

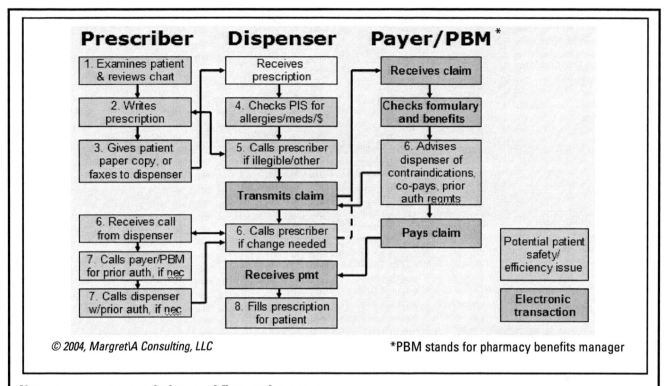

© 2004, Margret\A Consulting, LLC   *PBM stands for pharmacy benefits manager

Notes to current prescription workflow and processes
1. Medical and medication history is limited to what patient relates to prescriber, which may not include all medications or contraindications due to recall or restriction issues.
2. Prescriber's handwritten prescription may be illegible, incomplete, for a contraindicated drug, or written without knowledge of lower cost or more efficacious alternative.
3. Prescriber relies on patient to take prescription to dispenser.
4. Dispenser's knowledge of patient's allergies, medication history, and indications for drug is limited to that available from patient / retained in the pharmacy information system. (Although this may be more than what is available to prescriber!)
5. Calling dispenser to clarify prescription intent or discuss a potential lower cost or more efficacious alternative is time consuming for dispenser, prescriber, and patient.
6. When additional information is received from payer or PBM about contraindications to medications which the patient appears to be taking due to claims history, when there are issues associated with co-pays the patient can't afford, or when a prior authorization is required, dispenser must call prescriber to change prescription or obtain prior authorization—time consuming for all involved parties.
7. Prescriber calling payer/PBM for prior authorization is very time consuming, and can result in the prescriber making a change to another potentially less efficacious drug to avoid delay or cost to patient.
8. There is no direct feedback mechanism for the prescriber to know when the prescription is ultimately filled, partially filled, or not filled.
9. Dispenser calls or faxes prescriber for prescription renewal (additional refills) and prescriber calls/faxes back.

Steps six–eight: Identifying suitable workflow redesign and process changes, documenting the changes to submit to the system build team, and incorporating changes into policies and procedures are obviously the end results of the identification of opportunities and root causes. In the case of medication errors, studies have suggested that CPOE and electronic prescribing would significantly reduce medication-ordering errors and that bar code medication administration systems would significantly reduce medication administration errors. In this case, industry experts provided the answer to the problem. But it may not be so straightforward, even for your own medication ordering and administering systems. You may want to focus more specifically on individual tasks, or you may find that your vendor does not support bar code administration and you want to decide what other alternatives exist so you could make changes to reduce errors in this area.

For most other issues that are the focus of improvement opportunities, the solutions are not as readily apparent. This is where flowcharting current workflows and processes and formally analyzing them can be of immense help. Very often just listing the steps or drawing the diagrams provide for "ah ha" moments, as suggested in the description of Figure 5.3. In addition, having people on the team who are not performing the process on a day-to-day basis can help provide an "outsider's" perspective that can be invaluable. With little or no stake in the process, they will ensure that steps are not omitted from process considerations and can ask the tough questions.

As proposed workflows and process changes are suggested, it is important to document them. This not only helps to analyze them for their feasibility, but once consensus is achieved on the changes, they can be transmitted to the system build team and incorporated into proposed new policies and procedures.

Steps nine and 10: Not all new workflows and processes can be tested or trained on in advance of implementing the EHR. Where feasible, however, testing and training others on new workflows and processes serve two purposes. First, it helps determine whether the new workflows and processes are truly feasible. Second, it starts the change management process for other users, helps gain buy-in, and can help pinpoint unanticipated problems with the changes. Of course, an added benefit of actual implementation is that you can make improvements even without the EHR.

A word of caution here: Most changes are not completely feasible without the information technology support. Whatever changes can be made and do produce results should be attributed to the overall EHR implementation process. Many times, these improvements are not recognized unless planning for an EHR and would not have been done otherwise. Unfortunately, though, the EHR may not receive the "credit" for the accomplishment, potentially discrediting the full return on investment (ROI) for its implementation.

If it is not feasible to implement the new workflows and process changes, it is a good idea to use the documentation and proposed policies and procedures to introduce the changes to the user community. This can still initiate the change process and generate good ideas for potential modification. The ideas voiced from the full user community, however, should always go back to the workflow redesign and process change team to validate that the idea is not a response reflecting resistance to change.

Step 11: Obtaining pre-"go live" benchmark data to use in benefits realization studies is a step that may occur at multiple or different points within the quality and performance improvement process. Many organizations routinely conduct quality and performance data collection and can be the source for "before" data to use in comparison to data collected after implementation. If data are not routinely collected, data could have been obtained during step four to help identify potential opportunities for improvement. Some workflow redesign and process change teams, however, may be convinced of an opportunity for improvement even without such data. In this case, it is often desirable to start a data collection process so that you can determine results of implementing an EHR. Comparing pre- and post-"go live" results is formally known as a benefits realization study. Some organizations find this important—both for ensuring and celebrating success, and for documenting project results to executive decision-making bodies.

If a benefits realization study reveals less than desired results, the organization must look critically at ways to correct its course of action. It may be that there is less than desirable adoption of the changes and use of the EHR, that the proposed workflow and process changes are not as effective as anticipated, or that there is a problem with the EHR system causing a workaround that is taking away from its true potential for success. It is at this stage when the documentation of the initial assessment can also be helpful.

Step 12: Hopefully, the results of the EHR implementation are successful, and you can use the results of the benefits realization study for celebration. This may seem like we are jumping ahead to Chapter 10, which covers celebration of success and lessons learned. Although it is true that you want to celebrate at the "end" of the EHR implementation, an "end" to the implementation is often a long way off. It is important to celebrate success at every milestone achieved. But even though this step sets you up to do that at the conclusion of the EHR implementation, you should also do it each time a team turns over its plans for workflow redesign and process change.

Tools and techniques for conducting and documenting the assessment

There are a myriad of tools and techniques for conducting and documenting an assessment of potential quality and performance improvement opportunities and workflow redesign and process changes. Some are simple flowcharts or narrative aids that help identify steps in a process. Others are more sophisticated flow diagrams, sometimes automated, and sometimes accompanied by other supporting tools. Finally, there are a number of "management" tools typically used in one or more of the quality improvement methodologies identified in Figure 5.1. Some of these are statistical, others are diagrams of relationships, and still others are ways to help communications in workflow redesign and process change teams.

Simple flowcharts and narrative aids

A few simple flowcharts and narrative aids for conducting and documenting an assessment have already been identified:

- Benchmarking data is a very important tool. Healthcare organizations may be able to obtain benchmarks and best practices from a variety of sources, including state data reporting agencies, professional societies and associations, federal government programs, and others. In some cases, you may have to extrapolate the data from or used in conjunction with other measures.

- Flowcharts are simple to construct and easy to read. The advantage of the pictorial representation is to illustrate flow more clearly, especially where there may be decision points that generate branching. Figure 5.4 illustrates the symbols used to expand the flowchart to one illustrating decision points. Although these are easy to draw by hand, you can also construct flowcharts with most word processing and presentation software. For more elaborate flowcharts, use graphics software. Visio is a specific drawing software package from Microsoft that is frequently used to draw flowcharts, floor plans, and network diagrams.

- You can substitute step tables for a flowchart if you find pictorial representations of workflow and processes difficult to develop, or use them to analyze a flowchart, as illustrated in Figure 5.3. Step tables are more difficult to use where there is considerable branching, although not impossible. Figure 5.5 illustrates a step table and how you can incorporate branching. The figure also illustrates how to analyze each step. Step tables may be automated using spreadsheet software and can produce statistical graphs and analysis.

Figure 5.4 ▬▬▬▬ **Flowchart symbol usage** ▬▬▬▬▬▬

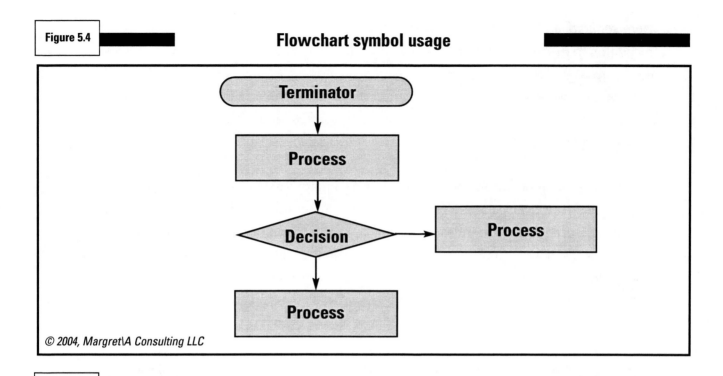

© 2004, Margret\A Consulting LLC

Figure 5.5 ▬▬▬▬ **Step table with branching** ▬▬▬▬▬▬

The following figure illustrates just the first few steps of a step table.

#	Condition	Step	Analysis
1		Examine patient and review chart	Medical and medication history is limited to what patient relates to prescriber, which may not include all medications or contraindications due to recall or restriction issues
2		Write prescription	Prescription may be incomplete, for a contraindicated drug, or written without knowledge of lower cost or more efficacious alternative
3	If	Patient is present in office and wants to take prescription to pharmacy	Prescriber relies on patient to take prescription to dispenser
	Then	Give prescription to patient	
	If	Patient is not present in office	Prescriber may make transcription errors if fax is unclear
	Then	Fax prescription to pharmacy	
4	If	Prescription is illegible	
	Then	Pharmacy calls prescriber	
	If	Prescription is legible	
	Then	Pharmacy checks for allergies, medication contraindications, and cost factors	Etc.

© 2004, Margret\A Consulting, LLC

More sophisticated/automated flow diagrams

In addition to the tools already illustrated, there are also "classic" flow process tools, meaning they are old but still useful. The flow process chart, such as the one illustrated in Figure 5.6, is an example. You may use the illustrated form to plot current steps in a process along with indicators for the type of action the step represents (e.g., operation, delay, storage). It also provides questions to analyze the steps and a place to record a revised process.

Although the intent of any quality and performance improvement effort is to reduce the overall number of steps and especially to reduce steps that do not contribute to the primary operations (i.e., the delays and transportations), new workflows and processes actually may introduce new steps. Such new steps, however, must contribute to the overall quality and productivity of the workflow and process. Remember, adding a step does not necessarily mean more time, but it could add time at one point in the workflow and reduce time downstream. Adding a step also may significantly enhance the quality of a given process if quality resulting from a flawed process is viewed as a problem.

For example, in sophisticated electronic prescribing systems, there are actually several additional steps the prescriber may take in the process of writing a prescription. The prescriber may more thoroughly review a patient's medical history if it is well organized and presented via the EHR. A more complete medication history may be provided through a payer/PBM consolidation service to which the prescriber subscribes. This may take a few additional seconds to check, or it could contribute data to the CDSS function, which provides more knowledge for selecting the most efficacious and cost-effective drug. Selecting all necessary attributes for the prescription may also take a few additional seconds. Finally, if the prescriber has the capability of checking eligibility, such a review could also add a few additional seconds or even minutes if patient counseling is required as a result. In total, the process of electronically writing the prescription may take noticeably longer than writing a prescription on a paper pad. However, the downstream time savings are potentially immense. Because the prescription is legible, more complete, and more accurate based on formulary and drug knowledge, you can nearly always avoid telephone tag with the dispenser, patient, and payer/PBM. In documenting such a before-and-after process, it is important to record all associated steps to illustrate the ultimate time savings and quality improvements.

Figure 5.6 **Flow process chart**

Process: ☐ Present ☐ Proposed ☐ Person ☐ Material								Analysis (✓):	Performed by: Date
Operation	Transportation	Inspection	Delay	Storage	Distance in feet	Quantity	Time		
								Why is it done this way?	
								Why is it done by this person?	
								Why is it done at this time?	
								Why is it done at this location?	
								Why is it done—is it necessary?	
								Details of Present/Proposed Process:	Notes:
●	→	☐	◆	▼				1.	
●	→	☐	◆	▼				2.	
●	→	☐	◆	▼				3.	
●	→	☐	◆	▼				4.	
●	→	☐	◆	▼				5.	
●	→	☐	◆	▼				6.	
●	→	☐	◆	▼				7.	
●	→	☐	◆	▼				8.	
●	→	☐	◆	▼				9.	
●	→	☐	◆	▼				10.	

Totals:									Present		Proposed		
								Summary:	No.	Time	No.	Time	
●								Operations					
	→							Transportations					
		☐						Inspections					
			◆					Delays					
				▼				Storages					
								Totals:					

Figure 5.7 ■ **Screen shot from BizFlow® for business process management and automated workflow** ■

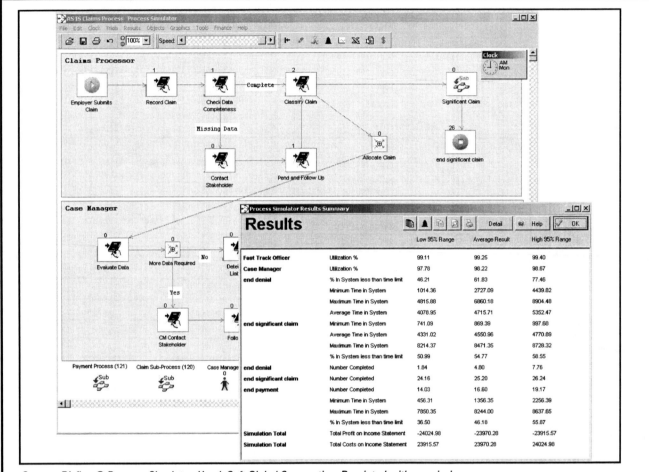

Source: Bizflow® Process Simulater, HandySoft Global Corporation. Reprinted with permission.

In addition to the classical flow process chart form, there are also automated tools that can provide similar and enhanced flow process analysis. BizFlow® by HandySoft is an example. It provides both flowcharting capabilities as well as tools to monitor workflow and volumes and to simulate changes. This tool is illustrated in Figure 5.7.

Management tools

As previously noted, management tools are derived from various quality improvement methodologies. They include statistical control charts as well as other diagrams. While none of these tools supply "answers" directly, they are designed to help workflow redesign and process change teams ask pertinent questions that will lead to better solutions. These tools are summarized in Figure 5.8.

Figure 5.8		Management tools	

Tool	Illustration	Purpose/Analysis
Pie chart		Used to show classes or groups of data in proportion to whole data set. Look for largest piece to find most common class. Look at relative sizes for unexpectedly similar or different sizes.
Bar chart		Used to compare classes or groups of data for both single and multiple categories. Look for the tallest bar, shortest bar, growth or shrinking of bars over time, one bar relative to another, change in bars representing the same category in different classes.
Run chart		Used to display process performance over time (events v. time period). Several variables can be tracked on a single chart. Look for peaks, valleys, upward or downward trends, and cycles.
Radar chart		Used to look at several different factors all related to one item. A point close to the center on any axis indicates a low value; a point near the edge is a high value. Look for average, minimum, and maximum alues in a series, the number of values in a series, the range, and the standard deviation that indicates how widely data are spread around the mean.
Scatter plots		Used to investigate possible relationship between two variables that are both related to the same event. A straight line (using least squares method) is included to identify best fit. Look for clusters that indicate positive (if x increases, y increases) or negative (if x increases, y increases) correlation. Note that correlation does not imply causality, but only potential relationship.
Histograms		A specialized type of bar chart that displays how frequently data in each class occur in the data set. Look at center and spread of distribution, as well as shape.
Pareto charts		A study of the distribution of events to identify the few vital factors that are causing most of a problem. Pareto was an Italian economist who proposed the 80/20 rule (that 80% of problems usually stem from 20% of causes.)

Figure 5.8 Management tools (cont.)

Normal test pilot		Used to investigate whether process data exhibit the standard "bell curve" and, if not, the extent to which processes are skewed.
Control chart (a.k.a. Shewhart chart)		Used to see variation in a process. Look for data points falling outside the control limits, whether points outside control limits are increasing or decreasing, and whether there are alternating up and down points.
Relations diagram		Show different relationships between factors, areas, or processes. Makes it easy to pick out the factors in a situation that are the ones driving other symptoms.
Cause & effect diagram (a.k.a. Ishikawa chart, Fishbone chart)		Used to explore all potential or real causes that result in a single effect. Causes are arranged according to their level of importance, resulting in a depiction of relationships and hierarchy of events in order to search for root causes, identify areas where they may be problems, and compare the relative importance of different causes. For service organizations, equipment, policies, procedures, and people are arranged in four major categories. Cause and effect diagrams can also be arranged as tree diagrams (see below).
Tree diagram		Used to determine all the various tasks that must be undertaken to achieve a given objective. It helps define the true scope of a project.
Affinity diagram (a.k.a., KJ method)		Used to discover meaningful groups of ideas within a raw list, usually derived from a brainstorming session. Ideas that seem to belong together are rapidly grouped, then ideas in question are clarified, and smaller sets that identify relationships are continuously sought.
Force field analysis		Used to build understanding of the forces that will drive and resist a proposed change. Two columns are used to identify driving and restraining forces. This is useful for analyzing factors that need to be addressed in change management.

© 2004, Margret\A Consulting, LLC

Change management

Change management is the effective management of a change such that executives, managers, and front line staff work in concert to successfully implement the needed process, technology, or organizational changes. Although described after the tools, it is not suggested that change management begins after workflow and process assessment. Rather, change management should start as soon as it is recognized that there could be potential changes—which is as soon as discussion begins about acquiring an EHR. Waiting until you select a place and are planning the implementation is too late because most staff members will "want to get on with it." The EHR is too big a project for it to go unnoticed by staff and others. If you are not straightforward with them and engage them along the way, they will be convinced you are hiding something and have every reason to distrust "establishment" and any proposed change. This is true for every type of organization, but it may be especially critical in a union environment. As long as the union is informed early and engaged throughout the planning and implementation, things will typically go much more smoothly.

Change perspectives

Critical elements for managing change include recognition of the fact that there are organization change management perspectives and individual change management perspectives. It is impossible to impose change from the top down without considering the impact of change on the individual. Likewise, it is impossible for the "rank and file" to accept change without support from executives and managers.

- Organization change management is the top-down component to change management that supplies strategies, communication plans, and training programs. Project mangers, project team members, human resources staff, and key business leaders/executive sponsors conduct organizational change management. For an EHR project, organizational change management is not only frequently accomplished through the EHR steering committee members and "super users," but also through physician and other clinician champions who help their peers understand and adopt the new technology.

- Individual change management is the management of change from the perspective of staff. They are the ones who ultimately must implement a change, such as using an EHR. The focus here is around tools and techniques to help the transition, such as from paper to electronic documentation or resource utilization. Coaching is required to help individuals understand their role and the decisions they make in the change process. Although project managers can provide tools that employees can use to navigate their way through the change, such as training programs, support staff during "go live," online help, prompts, and links to instructions, managers play a critical role in individual change management. A manager may not necessarily have been part of the EHR planning or implementation process, but he or she needs to be supportive of both the change itself and the process (and time) to adapt to change. With the cost and potential impact of the EHR-generated change program, non-supportive managers are often a detriment to success.

Model of successful change

Figure 5.9 depicts the ADKAR (Awareness, Desire, Knowledge, Ability, and Reinforcement) model , which is one way to achieve a successful change. These activities need to be timed so that they associate with the phases of EHR implementation: identification of the need for the EHR, conceptualization and design of the system, implementation, and post-implementation review and support. Unfortunately, many organizations fail to develop awareness early in the process and must jump into change at the point of implementation—which surprises staff, disrupts operational activities, and generally creates distrust throughout the organization. None of these are factors conducive to successful change.

Figure 5.9	ADKAR model of successful change

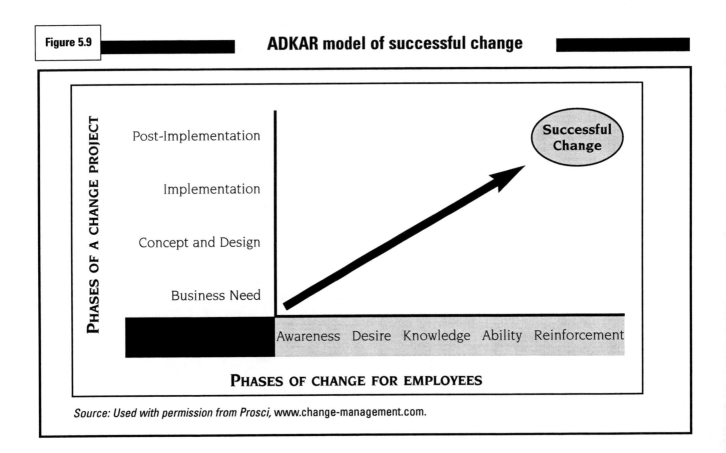

Source: Used with permission from Prosci, www.change-management.com.

Change management skills

Change management is not only about organizations and individuals and when to introduce change: Is about people who exhibit the skills necessary to lead change. Individuals who undertake change leadership positions need to have the following skills:

- Political skills—to understand, though not join in, the various viewpoints and counter viewpoints that may exist in the environment and how people may use them to achieve personal gain or support for their own group or cause.

- Analytical skills—to ensure that workflow and processes are not only understood and appropriately improved upon, but also to ensure the financial impact of the change. Few things speak louder than time and money.

- People skills—to understand the impact that change will have among all individuals, skill sets, and positions. Communication and interpersonal skills do more to achieve successful change than any tool or technique. Effective change managers are able to listen, restate, reflect, clarify without interrogating, draw out the quiet, quiet the verbose, channel discussion, plant ideas, and develop leadership.

- System skills—to organize and manage the technology and other activities associated with the arrangement of resources to produce specified results.

- Business skills—to understand the underlying way the company works or, in the healthcare organization, the underlying clinical processes. They need be able to "talk the talk" and "walk the walk."

Change management strategies

Although there is no "magic bullet" for achieving successful change, most effective change managers use a mix of strategies based on the degree of resistance to the impending change; the target population—whether large or small, professional or clerical; the stakes; the expected time frame; expertise of those affected by the change; and the level of dependency on people versus processes in the system being changed. These factors are then considered into one or more of the following strategies:

- Incentive-based strategy—is one in which conformance is rewarded. This is becoming more popular as payers have announced pay-for-performance incentives for providers to adopt EHR systems.

- Behavioral norm-based strategy—where behavioral norms or expectations are changed, either by organizational leadership or external factors. A good example is the promotion of bar code medication administration recently introduced by the JCAHO.

- Sanction-based strategy—may be viewed as the opposite of the incentive-based strategy, where nonconformance is penalized. In this case, payers may introduce disincentives. For example, Medicare has introduced additional time for payment on claims if not filed using the HIPAA-required electronic transactions.

- Adoption strategy—is one in which people are transferred from the old way to the new way over time. It may be that using the EHR is offered as an optional way of documentation. This strategy may be useful in some instances, but with the focus on clinical transformation (see below), most organizations find they do not have the time or resources for such a strategy. The strategy essentially requires running dual processes—paper records and electronic records. Such a strategy is extremely costly. (Note: A hybrid record environment is where the organization's official health record is composed of some paper-based documentation and some electronic documentation. For example, progress notes may be on paper but all results of diagnostic studies may exist only in the information system. A hybrid record environment may be a necessity based on information technology, but it is not the same as running dual systems where, for example, the diagnostic studies results are available in both electronic and paper forms.) As greater adoption of the EHR occurs, then management will ultimately be faced with a mandate to require use of EHR. Hopefully, individual benefits and peer pressure will often force the last remaining hold-outs to conform to the change before a mandate is forced upon them.

Practical change management tips

From a practical perspective and in summary, most successful change managers suggest that managing change is more a matter of leadership than of true management skill. Some tips from these successful people include the following:

- Fully engage yourself in the process. While you are leading, you must also be intimately involved.
- Have a clear sense of purpose, and do not waiver from that no matter how tough it gets.
- Build a team composed of people with the relevant skills and knowledge, but also with positive outlooks and high energy levels. Ask for volunteers.
- Maintain a flat organizational structure and rely on minimal and informal reporting requirements (while still ensuring documentation of all issues and factors directly impacting the new workflows and processes).

- Be action-oriented, flexible, and courteous. Recognize others for their knowledge and skills. Celebrate successes, draw upon lessons to be learned from failures, and never, ever blame or berate.

Clinical transformation

"Clinical transformation" is a new concept that has been introduced to describe the scope of change brought about by new health information technology (HIT) in general and EHR systems in particular. Regulatory, staffing, reimbursement, cost, malpractice, report cards, and other issues have catapulted organizations to seek a significant revamping of their workflows and processes to meet requirements, recruit and retain good staff, optimize reimbursement, reduce waste, reduce errors, and address public concerns. Clinical quality is now at the forefront of healthcare organizations' concerns.

For some consulting firms, "clinical transformation" has come to be a new buzzword to repackage old services, but true clinical transformation suggests some hallmarks that are different than previous approaches to change:

- Clinically focused—information technology prior to EHR and its various components has largely been on the periphery of the core business of health care—financial, administrative, and operational systems have been implemented. The EHR focuses directly on the core business of health care—taking care of patients—and the resulting clinical transformation programs have focused on the effectiveness and efficiency of patient care delivery.

- Integrated—where some of the financial, administrative, and operational systems were integrated or interfaced, often specialty or department-based systems were not linked to one another or to a core set of systems. To transform clinical processes, it is essential that all current and new systems serve as source, or feeder, systems linking directly or through a data repository to the EHR. Data sharing across all clinical systems is essential to the success of any clinical transformation process.

- Comprehensive—clinical transformation also relies on having access to all data for processing into the right presentation of information and clinical decision-making. Although many organizations go through a period of time in which they must operate with a hybrid record system, the goal is ultimately the ability to capture data from all sources for use in patient care delivery, management, and operations.

- Knowledge-based—clinicians are knowledge workers and demand that systems intended to support them be as knowledgeable as they. To date, hospital information systems or practice management systems have primarily addressed clerical and operational tasks. Although clinicians would be hard-pressed to function in an environment that did not have such systems, they are not touched directly by them as they are with clinical systems. If the clinical systems, however, operate in much the same manner—only supplying data back and not information based on solid evidence—they are of minimal value to the clinician. It is true that in some cases even availability of raw data did not exist with paper-based systems, but much more is expected, especially with respect to the actual cost outlay and human cost in adapting to change. Further, knowledge is continually evolving and changing. All organizations must recognize the EHR and, most particularly, the rules and alerts functionality are dynamic environments that must be continually assessed for accuracy and appropriately supported. It is only with this recognition and application of resource that utility of the system will remain at the highest levels of satisfaction and benefit to the healthcare organization.

- Outcome-oriented—clinical transformation is about achieving better outcomes. If there were a way to achieve better outcomes without major investments in information technology, these would be readily adopted. EHR systems, however, are recognized as significant contributors to improved outcomes. These investments not only must generate a ROI that is usually derived from reducing clerical and operational tasks, but they must continually prove themselves through better results.

Policy, procedure, and user manual development

As always, you need to document changes so they represent the policies and procedures of the organization. These policies and procedures are used in orienting and training new staff and also serve as the foundation against which results are benchmarked. User manuals provide specific instructions on use of the EHR. Although the EHR vendor may provide user manuals, any customization of the system performed by or for the organization will need to be reflected in the manuals.

Policies and procedures

Appendix A to this chapter provides guidance on policy and procedure development.

In short, policies are statements that establish goals of the organization. They provide guidance in making decisions about actions. Policies create mechanisms for detecting, resolving, and preventing violations.

Procedures describe how to carry out policies. They provide forms and formats for processing the operations associated with policies.

User manuals

For EHR systems, user manuals are often provided online. Ideally, they should work like an Internet search engine, where a user can key in any function, task, icon, or other element of the EHR about which they want to know and get specific help and directions. At a minimum, the online manuals should be highly indexed. Some manuals also have smart help where the system "knows" where the user is in a process and can direct help to that specific function.

If a user manual is provided in paper, it should be in a loose-leaf notebook so staff can easily insert updates. Again, the manual should be well-tabbed and indexed.

User manuals need to be kept up-to-date. Any change made to the system needs to be reflected in the user manual. This is as much a part of change control or configuration management (see Chapter 4) as common sense. Unfortunately, best intentions are not always achieved. Assigning someone to ensure that user manuals are kept up-to-date can help this.

Adding personal notes to user manuals should be a matter of organizational policy. User notes often reflect workarounds rather than true help in using the system as intended. For this reason, most organizations discourage users from adding notes to user manuals (and this is especially true for online versions). However, you also need a process by which users can submit questions and offer suggestions for improvement in those instances where user manual directions are not clear.

The goal of change

The goal of change is to improve. It is never to change just for the sake of change. Despite the fact that most organizations have no intention of making change to be disruptive, it is human nature to resist change and retreat to the familiar—at least to some extent. Some people can cope better with change than others. Even those who claim to thrive on change, however, often still want some comforts that the "old blanket" provides.

Clinical transformation is a good way to view the change brought about by an EHR. Clinical transformation is also a good way to express the need for an EHR. From either perspective, planning and managing the EHR workflow redesigns and process changes to achieve quality and performance improvements require the following:

- New visioning—that is clinically focused and directly related to producing higher quality of care and better outcomes
- New assessment—that is based on evidence that change is necessary and appropriate
- New engineering—that provides methods to rapidly reach solutions and that is sufficiently flexible to adapt to the dynamic environment that is health care
- New benefit analysis that ensures that intended results are achieved, lessons learned, and success celebrated

Workflow redesign and process changes feed directly into system build. Workflow redesign and process change activity generate the design of screens, determine which data is included in the structured entry templates, incorporate specific alerts and reminders, perform charting, and produce reports on a regular and ad hoc basis.

End notes

1. S.L. Strongwater and V. Pelote, *Clinical Process Redesign: A Facilitator's Guide* (Gaithersburg, MD: Aspen Publishers, Inc., 1996).

2. Institute for Safe Medication Practices, *The Five Rights*.

3. Institute of Medicine, *To Err is Human: Building a Safer Health System* (Washington, DC: National Academy Press, 1999).

4. A. L. Stewart, C. Sherbourne, R. D. Hays, et al., Summary and discussion of MOS measures. In A. L. Stewart&J. E. Ware (eds.), *Measuring functioning and well-being: The Medical Outcomes Study approach* (Durham, NC: Duke University Press, 1992), 345–371.

5. R. Kremsdorf, *The Five Rights of Effective Patient Care*, Five Rights Consulting, 2000. *www.informatics-review.com/thoughts/5rights/html*.

6. FCG for American Hospital Association and Federation of American Hospital, *Computerized Physician Order Entry: Costs, Benefits, and Challenges, A Case Study Approach* (January 2003) using data from Bates, et al., JAMA 274 (1995) 29–34.

7. W.L. Galanter, R.J. DiDomenico, and A. Polikaitis, "Focus: preventing exacerbation of an ADE with automated decision support," *Journal of Healthcare Information Management* 16, No. 4 (2002), 44–49.

Policy

Policies are statements that establish goals of the organization. They provide guidance in making decisions about actions. Policies are often based in law or other directives from regulatory and accrediting agencies. Policies create mechanisms for detecting, resolving, and preventing violations.

Procedure

Procedures describe how to carry out policies. They provide forms and formats for processing the operations associated with policies.

Creation process

In addition to using these templates, take an inventory of all policies and procedures currently existing in the provider setting. This will serve several purposes:

1. To identify policies and procedures that may already exist and should be modified based on the template content. This avoids duplication and confusion among members of the workforce who must follow the policies and carry out the procedures.
2. To identify where policies and procedures do not exist and need to be created from the templates.
3. To identify where policies and procedures exist that may be related to a required topic, but that are sufficiently different as to their need to be retired and replaced with new policies and procedures created from a template.
4. To identify policies and procedures that may be only peripherally related but that contain language that should be updated with HIPAA language.
5. To potentially identify existing policies and procedures that have not been followed and that require attention or special training.

Approval process

The volume of new and revised policies and procedures that the EHR generates may overwhelm the typical approval process in the organization. If this is believed to be the case, it may be necessary to take proactive steps to ensure that the requisite policies and procedures get approved on a timely basis.

Executive briefing

It may be appropriate to provide an executive briefing on the purpose, objectives, and focus of the EHR project immediately prior to the policy and procedure approval process. This will ensure full understanding of the scope of the EHR implementation and reinforce the context in which policies and procedures must be addressed. Such an executive briefing may remove misunderstanding relative to any individual policy and procedure and provide a more complete "package" approach to the approval process.

Executive sponsor

To that end, each policy and procedure, or group of policies and procedures, should have an executive sponsor. This executive sponsor should be made familiar with the policy and procedure to be sponsored so that (1) concerns can be raised in the drafting stage and (2) support will be garnered during the approval process.

Established process

Each organization has an established approval process. However, it may be worth adopting a modified process to "fast track" the EHR-related policies and procedures through approval, with the understanding that they are approved on a preliminary basis, subject to review within six to twelve months. This expedited review may reduce the number of steps and the tendency to achieve perfection.

Executive cover sheet

It may be appropriate to provide an executive cover sheet for each policy and procedure, or group of policies and procedures. This can serve to introduce the policy and procedure and may reduce or eliminate the need for full review of every document by every person in the approval process.

Executive cover sheet for policy and procedure approval

Policy name:	**Type:**
Number:	
Executive sponsor:	**Status:** ❑ New ❑ Revision **Date:**

Summary:
This is the essence of the policy and procedure in two to three sentences.

Impact:
Affected components: *Identifies classes of workers and/or departments most affected.*

■■■■■■■■■■ **Executive cover sheet for policy and procedure approval (cont.)** ■■■■■■■

Operations: *Highlights most critical elements that positively and/or negatively change the way the organization functions.*

Financial: *Identify operational and capital cash outlays required as well as any return on investment/loss avoidance that can be qualified.*

Risk assessment:

Briefly describes the risk of not implementing the policy and procedure, and the residential risk after implementation. (Risk may be described as high, medium, or low; or a formal risk analysis that rates probability of occurrence and impact may result in a numeric scale.)

Reason:

Describes why the policy and procedure is created/revised (such as the HIPAA standard being met). Should identify broadest scope of requirements addressed.

© 2004, Margret\A Consulting, LLC.

System Build

CHAPTER 6

System Build

The core technical process of implementing an EHR is the task of "system build." This is the most technically detailed task, and the one most specific to each vendor's product. This chapter focuses on the overall types of activities that encompass system build so steering committee members can understand them from a high-level perspective and the project manager can plan them. Actual technical details will have to follow specific vendor instructions.

In software development, system build is the process of converting source code into a machine-executable format that is run by the end user. In an EHR implementation process, system build is used in a broader sense. It refers to the myriad of changes made to an EHR product as necessary to fit the environment and potentially as desired by the end user. Some of these changes may result in source code changes. Most vendors can accommodate the need to customize the product through higher level processes that database administrators and data analysts can easily use. Some even allow users to tailor the system to their needs. System build capability is made possible by that fact that vendors design EHR systems to be flexible because they know each healthcare organization is different. This chapter

- promotes adoption of a configuration management strategy
- introduces the types of customization options available in most EHR systems
- describes steps needed to manage data successfully
- identifies typical user customization techniques
- provides resources for clinical decision support tools
- offers guidance on ensuring that EHR can support other healthcare and business functions
- summarizes technical controls that need to be managed during system build

Configuration management strategy

Before you or the vendor take any steps to change an EHR system, establish a configuration management strategy. Configuration management, sometimes called change control, refers to the tracking of changes in a system to ensure its integrity.

Modification v. customization

There are two primary ways in which changes are made to an EHR system:

- "Modification" is when the actual source code is modified to effect a change. Because modifications to source code alter the underlying structure of the product, many vendors do not want clients to do this. In some cases, such changes can nullify a contract. In other cases vendors permit modifications with certain clauses provided in the contract that put the onus of configuration management on the client in the event of incompatibility with future upgrades or versions. Vendors, however, may agree to do a modification of a product for a fee. Often the vendor will add desired changes by clients to a list of potential modifications that will contribute to an upgrade or new version of the product.

- "Customization," or tailoring, is when changes to the EHR application are designed for the client to make. The opportunity for customization may be minimal or extensive. In general, the more complex the system and the broader the vendor's target market for the EHR, the more flexibility will be built into the product. For example, the needs of a small physician's office are typically less complex than those of a large, multi-specialty clinic. As a result, the products sold to small practices may be limited in customization options. Similarly, the needs of a 100-bed community hospital would be less complex than those of an academic medical center or a multi-hospital integrated delivery network. An EHR product that is sold across the continuum of care will offer greater opportunity for tailoring than one targeted at a narrow slice of the market.

The process of customizing a highly flexible system to meet the needs and intended use in your environment is the primary definition of system build as described in this chapter. For complex products, this process can take months, or even years, to complete. Even for the least complex products, the process can take at least days, and often weeks. Performing system build for any EHR is much different than installing "shrink wrapped" software you buy at the local computer store for your desktop software. "Turn-key" EHR systems that require little building or allow little tailoring by the buyer are nearly extinct today.

Policies and procedures

Chapter 4 described configuration management as part of infrastructure preparation, and it included a sample policy and procedure in Appendix A. It is vital that you document any changes to the EHR and manage them carefully. The EHR encompasses clinical decision support with potential regulatory requirements for testing and certification with great impact on patients and their health outcomes; therefore, it is essential to have the ability to track changes. Figure 6.1 provides a simplistic example of the importance for maintaining system integrity.

Options selection

Another important component of the configuration management strategy is to determine the extent to which you will select and make and customizations. For some vendor products, customization tools

| Figure 6.1 | Example of maintaining system integrity |

A healthcare organization takes delivery of an EHR product that is version 2.3. It makes changes to the source code to accommodate user preferences.

At some future time, the vendor supplies an upgrade of the product to version 2.4. The healthcare organization may at this point make a decision to either ignore the (minor) upgrade or adopt the upgrade.

If the upgrade is ignored, track the fact that it was offered and the reason for ignoring it. Ignoring minor upgrades (those as indicated by change following the decimal point in a version number, such as from 2.3 to 2.4) could result in problems installing major upgrades (those as indicated by change preceding the decimal point in a version number, such as from 2.3 to 3.0).

If the organization decides to adopt the upgrade, it is essential that it understands what changes were made to 2.3 to determine whether and how those changes will impact 2.4. In some cases, there may be no impact and 2.3 can be upgraded directly with 2.4 while still preserving the changes made in 2.3. In other cases, the changes to 2.3 may have to be dealt with by technical systems analysts. There are a variety of ways to do this and development tools to support the process. The type of tools available depends on the platform on which the source code resides. From a philosophical perspective, a technical systems analyst may deal with the change by resetting 2.3 to its default structure, implementing 2.4, and then customizing 2.4 as necessary to incorporate desired changes as accommodated in 2.3. Having documentation concerning 2.3 changes is essential in understanding what changes to make to 2.4. Furthermore, whatever changes are made to 2.4 must be documented for the next change.

© 2004, Margret\A Consulting, LLC

are included; it is only then a matter of which options to build out. For other vendor products, it is up to the organization to determine the extent to which individuals, departments, specialties, or groups may customize the product.

What options

Part of selecting options occurs during the buying process when you decide what parts of the system to purchase. For example, an EHR vendor may offer optional applications to be used for computerized provider order entry (CPOE), electronic prescribing, medication administration, charting, clinical decision support systems (CDSS), patient care charting, interfaces to other vendors, personal health record components, etc. Your decision about whether to purchase each of these applications obviously has a huge impact on how you will use the system and how you will implement and build it.

You'll also make options selections within those parts of the system you did purchase. Examples of options might be which reports to use (many vendors offer far more reports than any one user would ever want to use), what rules from a CDSS to incorporate, what pathways or guidelines to incorporate to support patient care charting, etc. Even more detailed than this will be considerations concerning what vocabulary to incorporate, how much variability in screen layout the system will accept, and how much data analytics users may perform themselves. There may be literally hundreds of options to decide upon, many of which will have a huge impact on how you use your system.

Decision making

Obviously, these decisions, as well as others you make in the system build process, need to be well understood and carefully made. It is important that you have a logical and practical process for making such decisions. Some organizations attempt to establish an overarching policy concerning the nature and type of customization it will perform, or even let individual users or user groups perform. For example, some organizations permit individual physicians to create standard order sets, while others believe the downstream workflow and process issues from too many order sets is problematic and will only permit clinical departments to construct standard order sets. There are also standard of care issues that may dictate the source for clinical pathways, whether you will permit charting by exception, and the extent to which you must develop a rationale when users don't follow CDSS rules.

Because vendors typically design EHRs to be well-integrated systems, any decisions made about the EHR may also impact other decisions to be made down the line or by other departments for other systems within your organization. You must have a good understanding of how each option will affect the use of the overall set of systems in place. Typically, the best source of information for this is an experienced implementation person or support person from the vendor. You need to match that knowledge of the system needs with the knowledge and needs of your organization in order to make the right decisions. Thus, your decision-making process needs to incorporate vendor/product knowledge, along with user/organizational knowledge. This includes IT staff who will actually perform the customization working alongside those involved in workflow redesign and process improvement.

Management of data

One of the major areas in which customization occurs relates to how you manage data throughout the system. Data management includes selecting vocabulary standards and potentially mapping between vocabulary and code sets, creating or customizing tables, developing or tailoring data dictionaries, and managing the data repository, using a data warehouse, and providing data mining tools.

Vocabulary standards

The federal government has a number of initiatives underway to promote the adoption of vocabulary standards within EHR systems and other health information technology components. The Consolidated Healthcare Informatics Initiative (CHI) was expressly developed to get all government agencies that use health data to adopt a portfolio of existing health information interoperability standards (including health vocabulary and messaging) to enable all federal health enterprises to "speak the same language." Although there are 23 such federal health enterprises, which makes the task formidable, there could well be 23 different information systems in any given hospital that could conceivably use different vocabularies.

The National Committee on Vital and Health Statistics (NCVHS) was directed under the Health Insurance Portability and Accountability Act (HIPAA) to recommend uniform data standards for the electronic exchange of patient medical record information. It made recommendations for both interoperability (messaging) and vocabulary standards in July 2000, with several follow-up recommendations. These recommendations have been widely discussed and vendors are beginning to adopt them voluntarily. NCVHS was also tasked under the Medicare Prescription Drug, Improvement, and Modernization Act (MMA) to recommend standards for use in electronic prescribing. See *www.ncvhs.hhs.gov* for the full set of recommendations to the Secretary of the Department of Health and Human Services (HHS) on health data standards.

Another significant event for vocabulary standardization occurred when HHS licensed SNOMED-CT® so that it would be available to the industry free of charge through the National Library of Medicine

(NLM) Unified Medical Language System® (UMLS®) Metathesaurus®. SNOMED-CT® is perhaps the world's most comprehensive medical vocabulary, incorporating terms from many healthcare disciplines, including medical, nursing, and alternative care.

Efforts continue within the NLM to map various vocabularies and codes sets to preserve differences in vocabularies when possible and also coordinate the different vocabularies with other terms. For this purpose, SNOMED-RT® is used as a reference terminology. Figure 6.2 provides a diagram of the variety of vocabularies available and how the NLM has mapped them.

Figure 6.2   **Vocabulary mapping**

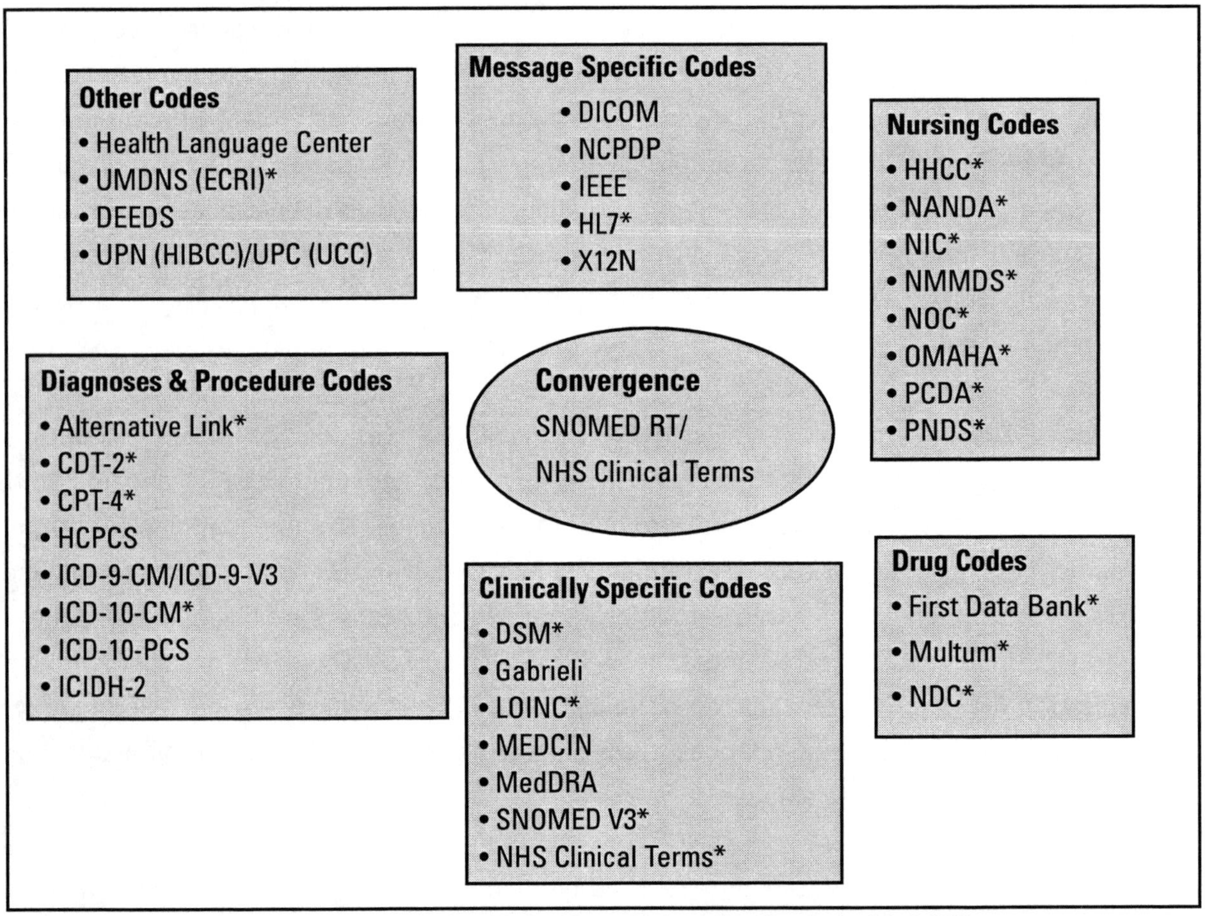

Other Codes
- Health Language Center
- UMDNS (ECRI)*
- DEEDS
- UPN (HIBCC)/UPC (UCC)

Message Specific Codes
- DICOM
- NCPDP
- IEEE
- HL7*
- X12N

Nursing Codes
- HHCC*
- NANDA*
- NIC*
- NMMDS*
- NOC*
- OMAHA*
- PCDA*
- PNDS*

Diagnoses & Procedure Codes
- Alternative Link*
- CDT-2*
- CPT-4*
- HCPCS
- ICD-9-CM/ICD-9-V3
- ICD-10-CM*
- ICD-10-PCS
- ICIDH-2

Convergence
SNOMED RT/
NHS Clinical Terms

Clinically Specific Codes
- DSM*
- Gabrieli
- LOINC*
- MEDCIN
- MedDRA
- SNOMED V3*
- NHS Clinical Terms*

Drug Codes
- First Data Bank*
- Multum*
- NDC*

Source: NCVHS Report to the Secretary on Patient Medical Record Information Standards, July 6, 2000.

What all of this means for the EHR, and for individual users of the EHR, is that you can construct data entry into the EHR to accommodate the capture of a highly diverse and medically robust set of discrete data. These discrete data can be shared seamlessly across different system components, can be mapped to other vocabularies and can maintain not only their syntax (structure and format) but also their semantics (meaning of terms), and can be used to support the rules that fire in CDSS. Use of standard vocabularies also enhance the capability of speech recognition systems to improve their accuracy rate, allow natural language processing to convert free text to discrete data, and to perform real-time data analysis—such as trending across disparate data (e.g., lab values against medications taken).

When buying an EHR system or other health information technology, look for incorporation of standard vocabularies. As the system is built out, it is also extremely important to retain the integrity of these vocabularies.

Database structure

Most EHR systems use some form of database to store and use data in a highly flexible manner. To facilitate openness and ease of integration with other systems, many vendors incorporate a database management system (DBMS) developed by one of the leading third party DBMS vendors, such as Oracle, Sybase, Microsoft, or IBM. Vendors create, define, and link the DBMS software products to the vast majority, and sometimes 100%, of all data elements to be stored in a database. To do otherwise would greatly increase the risk of customers adversely changing or damaging the integrity of the database, which could lead to serious errors in how the system performs.

DBMS are actually composed of a series of files or tables that together define the basic organization of the database. Most EHR systems use a form of database that is relational, where data are organized in a structure of related tables, each containing rows and columns. Figure 6.3 illustrates the table structure of a relational database.

In Figure 6.3, there are three tables illustrated. Each table has a relationship to one another, and potentially to (many) other tables. Within each table are various data elements.

Table development

One of the first steps in system build is to review all the tables supplied by the vendor to ensure that they reflect all types of data that the EHR needs to capture. Most EHR systems will have a relatively standard set of tables, which will reflect current standards of healthcare practice, such as tables for components of medical history taking, care planning, order writing, etc. The number of tables in an EHR will certainly number in the hundreds, if not the thousands. Although some vendor products

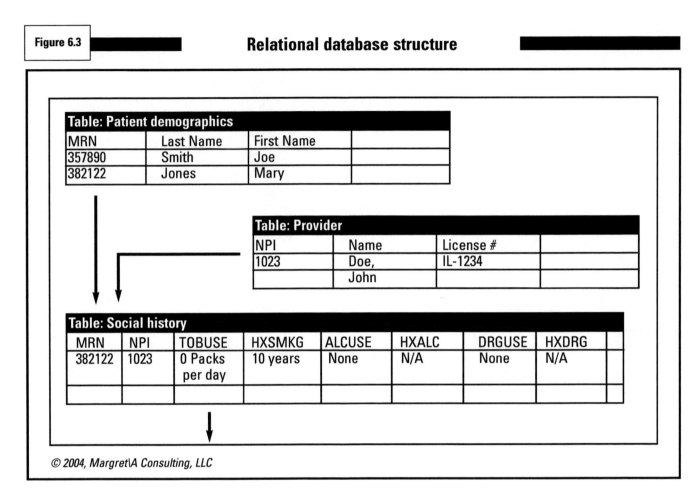

Figure 6.3 ■ **Relational database structure** ■

© 2004, Margret\A Consulting, LLC

permit the addition of tables, this is generally limited to specialty areas where the addition of tables will have minimal impact on the overall structure of the database. More commonly, vendors will tailor tables by adding, changing, or deleting data elements within the tables.

Master file tables

In addition to each individual table, Windows NT operating system uses a master file table (MFT) to keep information about every file and directory. It is a table of contents for the individual tables. If creating any new tables, it is pertinent for the database administrator (DBA) to update the MFT.

Data dictionary development

A data dictionary in its simplest form is a list of all data elements that the EHR must collect. When the EHR is based on a relational database structure (as most are), you may categorize the data elements by table, although very often the dictionaries themselves are databases that can be displayed in various sequences. In most EHR systems, the data dictionary serves as the key to describe all attributes of the data elements. A data dictionary that describes such attributes of the data elements is said to contain metadata (i.e., data about data). For example, if one data element that you want the EHR to capture is current tobacco use, the data dictionary would potentially include those elements listed in Figure 6.4. The data dictionary does not store actual data about a given patient, but it describes the data that it will collect and store about patients.

| Figure 6.4 | **Example of metadata in a data dictionary** |

Characteristics	Example
Name of entry	Current tobacco use
Table in which entry occurs	Social history
Physical name in database	TOBUSE
Synonyms	Smoker
Definition	Currently uses tobacco on a regular basis
Reference	AHRQ
Source of data	EHR
Derivations	N/A
Valid values	# packs per day
Conditionality	Mandatory
Default	None
Lexicon	SNOMED CTR®
Relationship	HXSMKG
Access restrictions	None
Process rules	Health maintenance: smoking cessation
Derivations	N/A

© 2004, Margret\A Consulting, LLC

As the example in Figure 6.4 shows, there will literally be thousands of data elements in a data dictionary. Every vendor will have its own form of data dictionary and specific metadata it records in the dictionary. Most vendors supply a "starter set" of data elements in a data dictionary. The organization then may choose to accept all the data elements in the starter set as supplied, or it may choose to review every data element carefully and make changes, additions, and deletions.

Suffice it to say, data dictionary compilation is extremely detailed. Due to the relationships between data elements, that they may be derived from computations performed on other data element values, and that they are used in clinical decision support rules, you must customize data dictionaries very carefully. Missing any one link can cause a significant downstream problem. How data elements are described in the data dictionary and then subsequently how they are displayed and processed in the EHR, however, have a great impact on users.

Although the data element in the example shown in Figure 6.4 is not derived ("Derivations" is marked N/A as not applicable), the value requires mandatory recording. This means that the clinician responsible for entering data into the "Social History" in the EHR is required to record some value. The "Valid values" is shown as "# packs per day," with no default values. This means that the clinician must enter some valid value. If the patient does not currently smoke, the clinician should enter 0, which would convert to "0 packs per day."

In some environments, perhaps those not focused on health maintenance activities, they could change this to an optional data element that the clinician could ignore. The default could continue to be none, so that the data element would contain no data, or it could be set to default to "0 packs per day." You can see that such a decision would have a great impact on clinician use of the system as well as the quality of data. After all, merely not asking a patient about current tobacco use or not recording an entry does not necessarily mean the patient does not smoke. It is also indicated in this data dictionary entry that this data element is used in a CDSS rule (i.e., "Process rules" identifies that the value is used in the "health maintenance" clinical decision support logic, under the component "smoking cessation"). The fact that someone else may depend on this data firing a rule obviously impacts its other attributes.

In addition to such attributes, the data dictionary specifies what lexicon (i.e., standard vocabulary, standard code set, proprietary list of terms) is used. Although a data dictionary can be comprised of proprietary data terms, most vendors are migrating to SNOMED CT® and various other complementary standard vocabularies that have been mapped to it.

Many vendors also set aside a small portion of their database for "user defined fields" or data elements. These are usually limited in number and often limited to specific uses to minimize the impact on the overall integrity of the database.

In evaluating potential changes to data elements in the data dictionary, an important factor to also consider is how to describe valid values. For example, "Current tobacco use" is described as having a relationship to "HXSMKG" (i.e., history of smoking). You could describe history of smoking in a variety of ways:

- Quit # years ago
- Occasional smoker
- Has smoked for # years

Each of these could need a description, such as for the individual who smoked occasionally for 20 years then quit five years ago. Although you can create a structured data entry capability to describe all of these factors, sometimes the level of effort in actually capturing this level of detail is more than the clinician wants to do. This may then be a target for an unstructured data field. However, clinicians must make such decisions, with the understanding of the impact to both their normal data capture processes and downstream use of the data. For example, if a health maintenance organization wants to conduct studies on the impact of smoking cession on other illnesses, it may be very important to collect a lot of structured data around this topic. Unstructured data will be much more difficult to work with.

Unstructured data

Data dictionary compilation focuses on data elements that need to record discrete data. Most EHR vendors find that clinicians also want the ability to enter unstructured, or narrative, data. Notice that in the data dictionary example in Figure 6.4, there is a relationship to another data element called HXSMKG (history of smoking). Current tobacco use and history of smoking are clearly different, as someone could have been a two-pack per day smoker until five years ago. Although it appears from the "relationship" entry that history of smoking is another structured data element, it is conceivable that the system would capture only current tobacco use in discrete data and a field left for recording variable data in unstructured, or narrative, form for history of smoking.

Because data values to be entered are highly variable, it makes sense to include some unstructured data recording capability. In some cases it is very difficult to anticipate what data values you will need to record for certain types of data. However, decision support rules can't process such unstructured data and will not necessarily comply with standard vocabularies.

Database management

Database management is a software tool that provides the structure to a database and manages the interrelationships among all the tables containing the actual data collected through use of the EHR. Database administrators (DBA) understand data-base management and are often used in larger organizations to continuously keep the table structures, data dictionary, and other aspects of the database current and in working order.

For example, when a code set is updated, such as when new ICD or CPT-4 codes are created, it must be incorporated into any processes that depends on "knowing" such codes. For example, if a code is added to CPT and that code could impact the level of service, it must adjust the relationship between those two data elements. In many cases, when a vendor supplies an upgrade, the upgrade is not only the new codes but addresses these relationships as well. However, it is possible that users may wish to make changes for which a DBA must make the relationships work as well.

Data repository

A data repository is a database with an open structure that is not dedicated to the software of any particular vendor or data supplier. Data contributed to a data repository come from diverse sources. They are stored so that you can achieve an integrated, multi-disciplinary view of the data.

A data repository may contain both discrete (structured) data and unstructured data and images. The images may be digital medical images, such as those from picture archiving and communication systems (PACS), document images where paper documents that have been scanned, as well as data that have been COLD (computer output to laser disk) fed from another information system. When presented to the user, data from a data repository appears as though it is coming all from one source. Such a screen will contain data that was entered as discrete data, may provide the ability to graph such data, will have data entry capability, and may include an icon or other marker indicating there is an image that the user can display as well. Clicking on that icon will cause the image to be retrieved into a window. It is not uncommon for a screen to look like the one illustrated in Figure 6.5.

Data repositories are typically sources for online transactions and often use the term "online transaction processing" (OLTP) to describe the fact that they interact with the user as requests are made to the repository for data or that data are sent to the repository once captured via the screen.

Figure 6.5 **Screen from multiple data sources in a data repository**

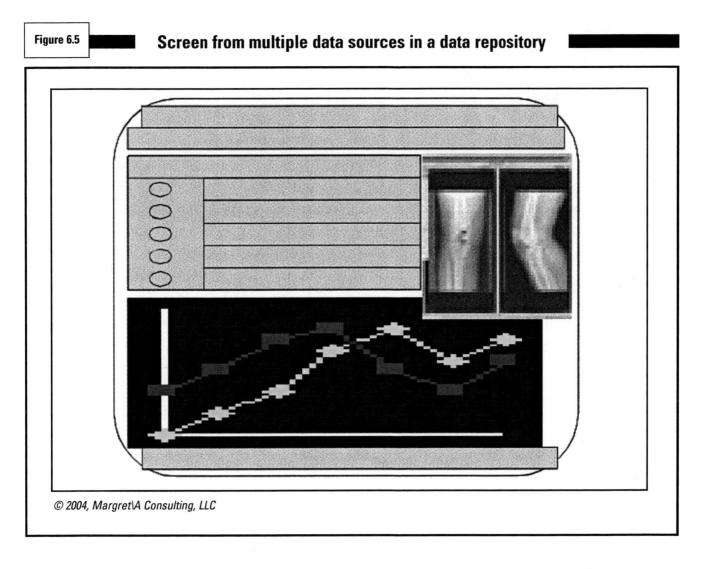

© 2004, Margret\A Consulting, LLC

Data warehouse

Because various analyses on data may take considerable amounts of data or very sophisticated computational processes, many organizations that perform such analyses will also develop another type of database, called a data warehouse. You can use the data warehouse to copy large amounts of data from the data repository for online analytical processing (OLAP). As a result, special analytical processing won't impact the performance of the data repository and its OLTP. A data warehouse in the context of EHR databases is not simply a place to archive data but to run complex analytical functions.

Data mining

Data mining is one of the analytical processes that a data warehouse typically supports. Data mining is the process of screening every data element in the data warehouse against specified criteria and extracting selected data, quantifying them, and filtering them to produce new information. Most end-users will not perform data mining, but they will be affected by it by virtue of having to record data in structured form.

User customization

Many of the system build activities prepare the EHR system for the user to directly use. For example, if in Figure 6.5, the graph were illustrating the impact of medication on certain lab values, the system build process would create the capability for the user to invoke graphing, select the variables to graph, and have the graph appear in a very short period of time (a matter of seconds).

Some systems, however, also include the ability for users to easily customize their own screens, create "favorite" views, rearrange lists of medications commonly ordered, etc. If the EHR is Windows based (i.e., uses a Windows operating system) and users are at all familiar with Windows, users should be able to drag and drop, set up preferences, reset colors, select optional views, and even recolor, size, and position various components of screen layouts.

As previously suggested, there are both positive and negative aspects to such user customization. It can be very helpful for a user to customize screens. It often makes user processes faster, contributing to better overall adoption. However, there are negative aspects of such customization as well. For example, if a user is able to create a "favorite" medication list, it is possible that new and improved medications may never make it to the list and could potentially limit the value of any medication decision support for which the overall system intended. Each organization needs to address the level of user customization permitted, and then set up the system so that users may only make those changes permitted. (It is generally not effective to prohibit customization by policy only, as skillful users will find a way to do what they want if not actually restricted.)

Clinical decision support

Much importance is given to clinical decision support in defining the EHR and establishing expectations for benefits from EHR systems. Many of the reasons behind structured data entry and compiling discrete data are to support clinical decision-making tools.

CDSS definition

A CDSS refers to the software necessary to build logical rules and generate alerts and reminders based on results of processing data through those rules. Rules can be as simple and helpful as offering tables and data elements specific to females when documenting a history and physical exam for a woman. Rules can also be highly complex, comparing the efficacy of various drugs against the patient's current medication list, conditions, and health plan benefits.

Types of clinical decision support

Generally, you can describe most forms of clinical decision support as one of the following:

- Alerts—those interventions provided by processing data through rules that identify a critical condition. The alert may be directed to a workstation in the form of red text, a flashing box, an exclamation mark, etc. You can program alerts to send a signal to a clinician's pager or even set off an alarm, such as in an intensive care unit. In general, healthcare organizations expect that alerts will be addressed with some form of action and documentation. This might be a simple act of turning it off, or a specific acknowledgement of the alert, required data entry, or other actions. Most, if not all, alerts should require some action.

- Reminders—are more subtle interventions. They may be the presentation of certain guidelines, such as described above for the female patient history and physical exam, or they may be notes that appear concerning the need to call a patient in for routine checkups, review of lab results, retesting, etc. Reminders might include the identification, through a hotlink, that there is reference material available relative to an entry made. This could be provided either in an unsolicited manner whenever a specific entry is made, or it could be a capability that is provided at the user's choice. Many organizations permit flexibility in responding to reminders.

Source of clinical decision support

There are a number of sources for CDSS, also called expert systems/rules. Most vendors supply a "starter set." These are basic rules most everyone buying an EHR desires. At the opposite end of the spectrum, users can develop their own clinical decision support rules and have in-house or vendor staff members write programs to have them run.

In between accepting what the EHR vendor supplies or creating your own, there are other sources for clinical decision support tools:

- Practice guidelines and clinical pathways available from medical and nursing specialty societies and the federal government's Agency for Healthcare Quality and Research (see *www.ahrq.gov*, National Guideline Clearinghouse®). Many of these guidelines appear "on paper" and need to be translated into computer instructions.

- Health plans also develop practice guidelines and generally make them available "on paper" or may support a Web site through which you can obtain guidance.

- Drug knowledge base vendors supply clinical decision support related to medication ordering with their products.

In addition to sources of guidelines, several companies develop third-party software to support clinical decision-making. They generally use standard vocabularies and incorporate evidence-based medical practice from research studies into algorithms for the support of rule-making.

There is also an HL7 standard for formal procedural language that represents medical algorithms in clinical information systems. The Arden Syntax encodes medical knowledge in a knowledge base form known as Medical Logic Modules (MLM). Each MLM is an "if-then" rule that executes a series of instructions, including queries, calculations, logic statements, and write-statements to generate clinical alerts and reminders. The Arden Syntax MLMs address interpretations, diagnoses, screening for clinical research studies, quality assurance functions, and administrative support.

Supporting other functions

The EHR is obviously a system that is designed primarily to support clinical patient care documentation and decision-making. But there are other healthcare aspects and business functions that the EHR needs to support. Additional healthcare functions extend the EHR beyond the "walls" of a facility to continuity of care, personal health care, and population health. Business functions include linking to charge capture and billing systems, the ability to produce business documents, executive decision support, and predictive modeling. Each of these important applications and modules needs to be built as part of the overall EHR system build.

Continuity of care

As more emphasis continues to be placed on providing care at the right level to reduce costs, patients receive care from many more provider types. This necessitates considerably more information flow between providers, and providers are finding that this is becoming a significantly greater burden than ever before. Reconciliation of medications, for instance, is an important issue across the continuum of care. Patient transfers from acute hospital to nursing home or home health requires considerable information. Making a referral from a family practitioner to a specialist, or among specialists is much more than sending a quick letter or making a phone call.

As a result of these needs, the ASTM International standards development organization, in conjunction with the Massachusetts Medical Society and several other medical specialty societies have created a continuity of care record (CCR) standard for data content to be used when referring patients. The CCR standard would permit transfer of data through electronic messaging systems, via a USB drive carried by the patient, or any other electronic, or even paper, means to exchange data. The standard defines what content is appropriate for sharing in the event of making a referral, transferring a patient care, and other scenarios.

EHR systems should be able to capture the data content in the CCR and supply it to whatever devices or means are used to exchange the data.

Personal health care

Many patients take it upon themselves to maintain their own personal health records (PHRs). In some cases, patients recognize that because they see so many different specialists, they must manage the flow of information among these providers themselves. Patients also use copies of discharge summaries, significant test results, patient instructions, and other documents to help them knowledgeably discuss their health conditions with their providers and to track appointments, vaccinations, and other wellness services.

Some patients understand the challenge of maintaining an accurate medication list at any given provider site. Under the pressure of illness and the healthcare encounter itself, patients know they may forget to tell a provider about a medication they are taking or not always recognize the importance of over-the-counter medications, herbal supplements, and others drugs. Their list of such medications, when they actually take them, what their response is, and when they may alter their medication regime or discontinue taking a medication on their own are facts that only patients themselves can describe for a provider.

In the past, providers were somewhat reluctant to accept such information compiled by patients, or "self-reported." However, many providers understand that this may be the only way to get a truly reliable history from a patient in certain situations.

Personal health records may be maintained in paper form at home, on an electronic device such as described for the CCR, via fax-back service, via an Internet service, or through a given provider's personal health record component to an EHR. An advanced EHR system should accommodate the collection and incorporation of PHR into the EHR system. Included in system build considerations would be determination of how to indicate source of data, managing reviews of those data by clinicians, the exchange of data when authorized, and the placement of restrictions as specified by patients.

Population health

Many new initiatives are being developed to address population health. Homeland Security programs have been one driver for this. Others, however, have included health plan and employer interest in disease management as well as public health departments' ongoing and ever-expanding roles relative to population health. International travel has brought many new conditions to countries never experiencing certain illnesses. International trade has introduced biologicals into countries' water supply and food sources that are not native and spread disease.

All of these factors contribute to the need for better reporting of data from EHR systems and better recognition of potential problems—often through advanced clinical decision support in EHRs that can recognize unusual symptoms, frequency of symptoms within a community, etc.

Business functions

Charge capture

Charge capture should be an obvious business function that an EHR must accommodate. This is a fundamental function, and system build activities must ensure its accuracy and completeness. There are also decision support functions that accommodate reimbursement coding, should ensure optimal coding, and spot the potential for coding that could be considered fraudulent or abusive.

Business documents

The ability to produce business documents, however, is an often overlooked function of an EHR. In fact, the inability to produce paper documents representative of the content of the health record has led to at least one vendor claiming—"why print? This is an electronic record!" However, there will continue to be a need to print documents for various release of information purposes, including response to subpoenas and court orders. In addition, many healthcare organizations do not give up their paper record systems despite maintaining an EHR. In this case, paper records can balloon in size as a result of having to print every screen. Although ideally the paper records should be done away with, there are other issues associated with retrieval as well. Being familiar with the format and structure of paper records, auditors and others who perform quality improvement activities, revenue cycle management, clinical research, and other clinical but non-patient care tasks may find it difficult to navigate through an EHR that is essentially designed to document and fire decision support rules. Retrieval strategies should be considered at least one component to system build.

Registries

Registries are yet another potential use of data that the EHR must manage as part of designing data capture and data management strategies. Formal registries include cancer registries, cardiac registries, medical device registries, and others. Data sets ar e not her important factor. An EHR must accommodate the need to contribute to state data registries or for other licensing and accrediting activities, such as JCAHO's ORYX and NCQA's HEDIS data collection programs.

Executive decision support

Likewise, the EHR must also accommodate executive decision support—the ability to use aggregate data to monitor clinical trends for marketing and other business planning activities. For example, when you make decisions about what data should be structured, you need to understand the type of data executive decision makers need.

Predictive modeling

Finally, predictive modeling is a fairly new science in which data are used in sophisticated computation processes to supply new clinical practice guidelines in general and to predict the potential for disease in individuals in particular. Once again, how data are captured and managed in data repositories are important elements in the ability to perform predictive modeling if healthcare organizations intend to do so.

Technical controls

Technical controls are a final consideration in system build. Technical controls refer to various security measures as well as data integrity and accountability measures.

You can use the HIPAA standards as a source document for understanding what security controls you should implement in an EHR system. However, there are two important considerations in EHR system build relative to technical controls:

- Implementing stronger controls than what have typically been available for departmental or source systems is generally a requirement in an EHR system. By far, more sensitive data are captured and many more users may have access to such a system. Strict enforcement of unique user identification and authentication measures is critical for an EHR. In addition, access controls are needed that ensure access to information for treatment but restrict access where there is no treatment relationship. These include quick and easy emergency access procedures ("break-the-glass") and audit trails. Consider encryption and digital signatures especially as data are shared across the continuum of care with other providers and as clinical users begin using more hand-held, wireless devices and remote access. CCRs and PHRs need appropriate controls for both patients and providers, including accountability of the data entered or retrieved, as well as integrity controls relative to what changes were made.

- Ensuring that controls are persistent throughout a system build, upgrades, and other changes. Because system build activities—whether for new systems or upgrades—often require resetting to default modes, security measures may be temporarily turned off. Even though the intent may be true only for the test environment, it is not uncommon for such defaults to not be reset in the haste of providing the new system functionality to users. Automated configuration management controls can help considerably in ensuring that you address these technical controls. If such aids are not available, you must enforce strict adherence to configuration management policies.

Good news/bad news

System build is both the good news and the bad news relative to EHR implementation. System build helps make an enormously complex system intuitively available to end users. Alternatively, system build takes a huge amount of time and an enormous level of attention to detail. If such time or attention is not available, it is generally better to avoid getting too deep into customization and leave changes to the vendor at the time of system upgrade. If available, however, it is extremely rewarding to create a system that precisely meets your organization's needs—and it pays off in heightened adoption of the system and the resultant benefits.

CHAPTER 7

EHR Testing

CHAPTER 7

EHR Testing

Testing is the process used to verify that the EHR works as intended. As you prepare the technical infrastructure and accomplish process redesign and system build, you must ensure that testing is performed. Not only do you want to know that all the components of the system work, but you have a contractual obligation to determine that they work as described. However, as suggested in Chapter 3, aspects of EHR implementation are not performed solely in a sequential manner. As such, successful testing is generally considered the concluding element of each phase of implementation, including but not limited to the last phase. A good way to look at the timing of testing is to consider testing (and remediation and retesting as necessary) the step immediately before each milestone on your project plan. This chapter

- emphasizes the critical importance of thoroughly testing the EHR
- identifies the levels of testing typically needed for an EHR
- offers suggestions on how to conduct tests of the EHR
- describes how to establish a test environment for the EHR
- provides practical advice on achieving a properly working EHR system

Importance of testing

There are strong business, clinical, and legal reasons for thoroughly testing any information system that is acquired. This is especially true for EHR systems due to their complexity, clinical nature, and interdependencies with other systems.

Business reasons

From a business perspective, you need to ensure that the product you implement is delivering what you expected it to—i.e., that you are getting what you paid for. It is impossible to expect that the benefits of an EHR can accrue if there are faults in the system. These must be repaired prior to moving forward. Because the EHR so directly impacts clinicians who may not have used computer systems in the past, testing the outcomes of their use is critical. There have been significant failures when organizations implement systems without adequate planning, workflow redesign and process change, and training for users. A failure costs an organization not only in wasted financial and human resources, but often in the ability to move forward with other information systems projects. For example, a failed CPOE system can dramatically impact whether a nursing documentation system may be successful as it will fuel skepticism and more resistance to change.

Clinical reasons

Clinical reasons for testing the EHR are of great importance because the EHR may have a direct impact on the well being of the patient.

In addition to the obligation of a provider to ensure quality health care, government/regulatory agencies may require evidence that you have adequately and successfully tested the system. For example, the Food and Drug Administration (FDA) already has requirements in place that must be met for certain clinical systems, such as a blood bank system. These systems may be part of your EHR or interfaced to it. In fact, the FDA also has regulations regarding testing of any system that has a clinical decision-making component to it. Although the FDA may not yet have invoked these regulations with respect to EHRs, there is always the possibility that they could.

Accreditation agencies, such as JCAHO, may include review of newly implemented systems in their accreditation reviews. They will certainly look at them to ensure that their standards for information management are met and its impact on the quality of care rendered.

You can expect that external requirements for EHR testing will increase over time. Payers are starting to implement pay-for-performance systems where the ability to produce data on outcomes is necessary for the incentive. Without an EHR, it is virtually impossible to collect the data to be reported for a pay for performance system, or it least recoup the cost of data collection in a manual mode. Regulatory reviews or data collection requirements will not only require you to test the system thoroughly, but possibly to produce documentation providing legal evidence that you have done the testing.

Legal reasons

Contractual terms supply the legal requirement for testing. The contract for acquiring the EHR software defines your rights and obligations to test as well as defines the vendor's obligations and limitations concerning the validity and integrity of the tested system. You need to identify any problems, flaws, or issues with the EHR as soon as possible and well before using it for actual productive use. Your vendor shares the same intent, but it also wants to get the EHR implementation "finished" as quickly as possible to minimize effort and cost. The vendor also wants to get paid in full for the system. In fact, a good contract should tie (a final) payment for the EHR to successful completion of testing.

As a side note: The difference in incentives for buyer and seller makes it critical that the buyer conduct testing. As a prudent buyer, you need to take ownership of the entire testing process, develop test plans and tools, and execute them on your own terms. To be sure, the vendor will need to support and perhaps provide some guidance to the testing. As the saying goes, however, you need to be sure you don't hire the fox to guard the hen house.

Types of testing

Testing parallels the psychological principle of Gestalt—"the whole is greater than the sum of its parts." Simply put, this means that you need to validate that each component, module, and application that encompasses the EHR works as designed and expected. Figure 7.1 illustrates these parts as used in the testing activity.

Figure 7.1　　**EHR parts**

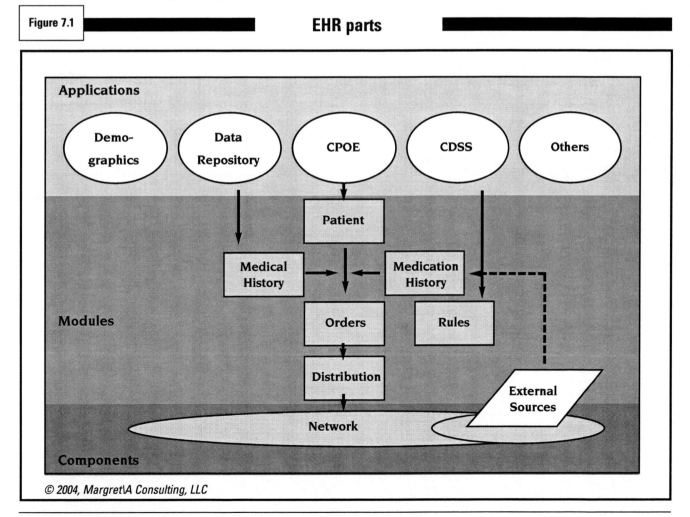

© 2004, Margret\A Consulting, LLC

- Applications refer to the logical parts of the system that are often sold separately. These may include a data repository, clinical decision support system, CPOE, patient care documentation, or any other feeder systems necessary to fully capture all data needed for patient care.

- Modules typically refer to logical parts of an application. For example, in a CPOE application, there will be demographic data feeds to associate the order with the patient, medication history that may come from an external claims source,1 the actual order, rules that may fire about the order such as an allergy alert or a reminder to check certain lab results, and the distribution of the parts of the order to pharmacy, lab, dietary, etc.

- Consider components as the infrastructure elements, such as network connections, human-computer interface devices, data conversion, etc. necessary to use the EHR.

Each collective part of the EHR system results in several layers of testing. Although test phases and methodologies will vary by vendor and preferred approaches, they typically include the layers illustrated in Figure 7.2.

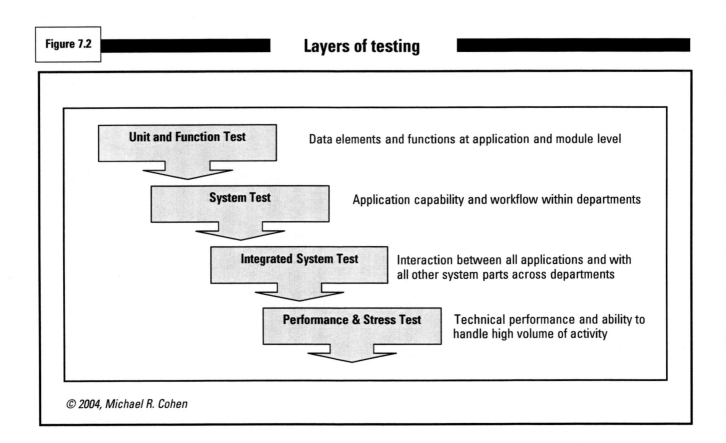

Figure 7.2   **Layers of testing**

Unit and Function Test   Data elements and functions at application and module level

System Test   Application capability and workflow within departments

Integrated System Test   Interaction between all applications and with all other system parts across departments

Performance & Stress Test   Technical performance and ability to handle high volume of activity

© 2004, Michael R. Cohen

Unit and function testing

Unit testing focuses on validating that every data element in the system has been built/defined properly and works properly. Frequently, it is also used in the broader sense to include what some refer to as functional testing—which is intended to validate that each individual function within the system works properly. Both are typically conducted at the application and module parts of the system. For example, if the EHR is comprised of multiple applications, such as a nursing application, a CPOE application, etc., you would conduct tests separately for each of the applications and potentially for each of the modules within the applications.

The key to unit and function testing is thoroughness—it is essential that every important function and data element be tested at this level. Although subsequent levels of testing may also catch some errors at the function and data level, it is not their intent to do so. If such an error makes it through unit testing, there is a good chance you won't discover it until you are using the system in a live environment. Once in production, a system error could have a disastrous effect. For example, if a correction a nurse made in recording vital signs does not display properly, it could result in a physician decision to increase medication dosage to a level that is clinically unwarranted.

Such thoroughness requires testers to develop a comprehensive plan that documents all the functions and data elements to be tested, records the results of each test, and provides the means to communicate errors or problems to the vendor responsible for fixing them. Figure 7.3 provides examples of items to include in your unit and function-testing plan.

Unit and function-testing plan

Unit and function testing entails testing the following:

- All major functions. Use a comprehensive list of all functions performed by the EHR. Because most vendor contracts stipulate that "what you are buying is the system as defined in their system/user manuals," it is a good idea to use such documentation as a basis for testing.
- All design changes/requests made for the application. Such "customs changes" are among the highest risk components of a purchased system.
- Every screen. Every screen needs to appear as expected, including checking the elements listed below. In many purchased systems, this is partially controlled by the buyer through the use of tailoring tools provided by the vendor. Hence, it is important to keep track of such design changes/tailoring made by the organization.
  - ◆ Content, fields, codes, dropdowns, messages
  - ◆ Spelling
  - ◆ Field edits (for value, required/optional/descriptive, etc.)
  - ◆ Flow as expected
- Every data element. Check every data element and especially those elements you have added or modified for
  - ◆ spelling
  - ◆ definition and use
  - ◆ acceptable values (many of these are built by the user; e.g., physician names, valid beds, specific names (and mnemonics/codes) for any item that can be ordered, etc.)
- Clinical alerts and reminders. Test that every clinical rule triggers the appropriate alert or reminder under the designated set of circumstances. For example, if you have built a rule such as "Upon entry of Bactrim DS in CPOE, check urinalysis that Bactrim DS is appropriate for the specific organism," then a test should be run for various scenarios in which Bactrim DS is ordered.

System testing

System testing validates workflow and system use within a single department or application. System testing should include testing processes that require sending or receiving information to other departments and applications, including ensuring that interfaces pass data correctly from one system to another. For example, a medication order should result in data being sent from the CPOE application to the pharmacy, nursing, and other areas. As part of system testing, the group responsible for testing orders would want to ensure that the order was properly sent to and received by these other

---

areas. Because this stage focuses just on this specific application or department, however, this test would not be concerned with what happens to the order after it is properly received by the other areas.

Because most workflows typically involve many steps and "handoffs" of data from one person to another, it is best to develop and use "test scripts." These scripts will define realistic examples of actual patient/process scenarios experienced in your organization. Figure 7.4 provides an example of a test script.

Figure 7.4	**System test script**

Test script for CPOE application

- Physician orders Penicillin for patient
- Prior patient history (which would need to be entered prior to test) includes an allergy to Penicillin
- System flags potential serious allergy interaction and alerts physician
- System recommends potential alternative medications
- Physician searches patient file for additional patient information
- Physician orders alternate medication
- Order sent to applicable areas

© 2004, Michael R. Cohen.

Scripts should include all major processes. Each step in the script should indicate who is responsible (i.e., nurse, clerk, physician, etc.) for that step in the work flow, specific information that needs to be entered, what the expected results of the step should be, and whether each step passed or failed the test.

Integrated system testing

After earlier tests have validated the data elements, functions, and work flow/system flow of each application, you will be ready for integrated systems testing. The intent here is to simulate the "live" environment and ensure that all the applications, modules, and components of the system interact according to design and expectations.

Because this is usually the "dress rehearsal" before "go-live," you should achieve the following objectives:

- Ensure all system parts (EHR and interfaced systems) that share data or depend on other parts work together properly.

- Ensure that patient data flows properly through the system.

- Ensure that users know how to interact properly with the system and that user procedures work properly. This is an excellent place to reinforce user training. It is also the time to fine-tune policies, procedures, and workflows.

- Ensure that all input, processes, workflows, and output work as designed. Although these have been thoroughly tested in earlier stages of testing, include mission critical and higher risk functions in the test. Figure 7.5 provides examples.

- Discover, diagnose, and fix those items that do not work properly.

The list in Figure 7.5 is by far the most complex layer of testing to plan, orchestrate, and conduct. It should involve a cross section of staff from all departments and applications in the EHR, including those systems with which the ERH interfaces. Although it is usually the "super-users" and "core team" players who are most involved with this level of testing, it is highly desirable to get additional users,

---

Figure 7.5 ▮ **Examples of mission critical and high-risk functional tests** ▮

Test situations requiring:

- Complex logic, such as 24-hour observation, Medicare readmit
- Clinical logic, such as drug/drug, drug/lab, drug/food interactions
- Complex calculations, such as pediatric drug dosage
- Known pain points with current system or current processes and workflows
- Newly designed, major processes and workflows
- Exception logic
- Clinical alerts and reminders
- Many departments, positions, and people to "pass the baton," especially where there are known problems in current processes and workflow

© 2004, Michael R. Cohen

---

trainers, and clinicians involved, as well as IT staff. There are two reasons for not relying exclusively on the core team. First, it is an excellent platform for reinforcing/validating user training. Second, users who are not quite as familiar as the core team would be less likely to take short cuts and may have subtle differences in how they use the system that wind up exposing potential weaknesses.

As in system testing, the primary tool used for conducting the test is the test script. In fact, where practical, you can build upon the system test scripts to create the more comprehensive integration system testing scripts. To more fully test the reality of the system, these scripts typically involve multiple day scenarios. Figure 7.6 is an example of such a script.

Figure 7.6	Multi-day integrated system test script

Test all transactions for:

Day one: Patient admission, diagnostic studies ordered and conducted, and preliminary diagnosis made.

Day two: Based on the results of diagnostic studies, course of treatment is defined and additional orders placed.

On both days, clinicians would take notes, track progress, view reports, etc. These actions would trigger other transactions, such as charge capture. As data is shared among applications, it would invoke interfaces with other systems, such as diagnostic lab equipment and clinical systems from other vendors.

Day of discharge: Test all discharge processes.

© 2004, Michael R. Cohen

Keep in mind it is not practical to test every function and data element in integration testing—that is what earlier stages of testing are for. However, there should be a sufficiently large number of scenarios to ensure that all major processes and all hand-offs of information are fully tested. You may need to test anywhere from 25–100 scripts, of varying size and complexity, for a comprehensive EHR system. During the actual test, the entire test team might be in one large room outfitted with all the necessary computer equipment, peripheral devices, and supplies to support the test. Each person/department listed on each script would then conduct their respective part of the test in sequence. Each part might only require a few minutes of time entering information. But you must scrutinize the results to ensure that everything works as expected. Note all results of the tests—both positive and negative—on the script, along with the testers name/initials. If any part of the test is not successful, you should repeat it to try to replicate the error. If you can't replicate an error or problem, it may either not be an error or may be an insidious kind of error that occurs only under the most unusual circumstances. In such a case, you should keep trying to replicate the error until you are convinced either that it is not an error or that it is not identifiable. If you do replicate the error, you must escalate it to the point where you can track and correct it. A decision then needs to be made as to whether the error prevents the rest of the script from being tested at that time or not.

As each person is done with a part, the script is handed off to the next person on the script, representing the next step in the process flow. A good script will be handed off many times during the test.

It is not unusual to experience "script errors," where someone performing a test part is unable to complete the part because the information needed or some predecessor part has not been done (since it was not scripted). The realistic accuracy, thoroughness of testing, and reduction of scripts errors is best achieved by having the scripts developed by multidisciplinary groups crossing all departments, applications, and positions affected by the EHR.

Due to the importance and complexity of integration testing, as well as for the need to fix and retest errors that have been found, integration testing is often conducted in two or more sequential sets. The "final" round is the last dress rehearsal, and if the system "passes the test," the system is ready for conversion to "go-live" status, as long as all other necessary conditions are also ready. For this reason, vendors sometimes refer to the final round of integration testing as the "final acceptance test," which may trigger a significant milestone and payments that may be tied to that milestone.

Performance and stress testing

Performance and stress testing are focused on validating that, from a technical and operational point of view, the system is able to meet the real demands of "live" use. For example, performance testing would measure response times for key transactions or interactions with the system and ensure they are within acceptable limits, which may be defined in the contract. It would also include validating that the configuration of the central equipment, remote equipment, peripheral devices, network, etc., work properly under simulated conditions.

One of the conditions to be simulated, referred to as stress testing, is to create an extremely high volume of activity on the system at the same time. Ideally, this would exceed anticipated peak loads of system usage, to provide you some margin of error that the system will meet your needs during actual periods of high use. This is a much more technically oriented form of testing that requires heavy involvement from system architects, network managers, database administrators, operations managers, and other highly skilled technical professionals from both the client and the vendor organization.

Some suggest doing performance and stress testing prior to integrated system testing. The idea here is that additional infrastructure may have an impact on the totality of the system functionality. However, doing performance and stress testing prior to integrated system testing will not reflect the changes made to the functionality—such that performance and stress testing may have to be performed again. In very large EHR implementation, some of these tests may need to be run in parallel. However, most organizations find they need to have a full set of functionality in place and working before a final determination can be made on load.

Test environment

As the examples above illustrate, it is necessary to have a closely controlled test environment, including a test database. Define and maintain the test database according to an agreed upon test plan. Develop the test database as the system build for the application is nearing completion. Obviously, it is not complete until testing validates that it is ready, but starting too early can be a futile exercise in having pieces of the test fail simply because they were not built yet.

Other aspects of the test environment include ensuring that there are separate components on which to run the test that do not impact the production system. While various applications, modules, and components of the EHR are being tested, many day-to-day operations are being performed and cannot be disrupted because a test of the EHR caused a component failure.

The test environment also includes persons specified to participate, the test scripts developed, the documentation of the tests, and the process used to resolve issues identified during the tests.

Testing practicalities

EHR testing is difficult and has high stakes. This testing must validate that a very expensive system will perform as expected. Once the EHR is deemed to have passed all forms of testing and is converted to live status, two important cultural and economic events occur. First, the system will create a huge (and hopefully positive) impact on the organization. A positive impact can ensure achievement of many benefits. A negative impact can be catastrophic to the organization and the implementation team. Second, your vendor probably will have received final payment (unless you are able to withhold a significant portion until some time after go-live). With that last payment, you lose leverage in having the vendor fix problems, especially since it was up to your organization to find them earlier and it failed to do so.

As a result of the enormous impact of the EHR, it is important to establish appropriate accountability, keep good records, and use a formal issues management structure.

Accountability

A simple method used to establish accountability is to require testers/departments/key users to sign a form acknowledging that they have conducted a thorough test and certify that the system has passed, perhaps noting any specific concerns or failures as appropriate. Some organizations require such sign off for each testing level, others only after final integrated system testing. But assuming accountability in this formal matter puts the onus on the individuals to do the very best they can on the testing process. Each individual assumes accountability for a part, rather than attempting to pass accountability to another person, the IT department, or the vendor.

Documentation

It is very important to keep written records that can demonstrate the testing that has been done, describes how well the system performed during the tests, and identifies any detected errors. These records need to be easily recoverable in case they are needed as documentary evidence of your efforts. As mentioned earlier, there may be government or regulatory agencies asking for evidence of your testing, perhaps as far in the future as 10 years after the system is implemented. More likely, however, is the internal need for them. Internal needs include the ability to deal with questions or issues arising in later testing or after go-live. Such questions or issues might include: problems that were identified, but were not fixed satisfactorily; problems that occurred later that someone could claim should have been discovered but were not; or problems that appear to have arisen due to subsequent changes or updates, but were not problems at the time the system was accepted. Documentary evidence can be very powerful in building or protecting your case for fixing such problems. The lack of documentary evidence will create an easy area for potential adversaries to exploit.

Issues management

How often in life are you given a chance to try to break something and get praised if you find a problem? It is good to find errors during the testing process. You want your tests to be tough and thorough so whatever problems exist will be found at this point and not during normal use. Using a baseball analogy, during batting practice, you don't want to pitch *as though* it is batting practice, giving the hitters an easy time hitting that 420-foot homerun. Instead, you want to throw your best stuff at them—the 98 mph fastball or sweeping curveball—and make them fail as often as you can so they will have worked on everything by game time.

Equally important to finding errors and problems is having a process in place to track them. This includes describing the problem, giving evidence and documentation that vendors can use o diagnose and resolve, assign accountability to fix the problem, and track it through resolution. Once a problem is deemed corrected, you need to retest it.

Besides error correction, changes in the EHR being implemented can be many and frequent. Track these changes to ensure that their impact is understood and to determine when and whether you need to retest the system with those changes. Sources of such changes might include specific requests made to the vendor, changing profiles or options on the system to "tweak" it, new releases and versions implemented by the vendor, and changes implemented by third-party vendors (e.g., a Microsoft Windows XP change that inadvertently affects the system). It is critical that you manage these changes, especially late in the implementation, to avoid unpleasant surprises where a change adversely affects some aspect of the system. During the system build process there may be "domain refreshes" that put all changes out at once. Retest the system after each refresh or after any other major changes, a process referred to by some as regression testing.

Stress of testing

In addition to stress tests on the EHR system itself, testing itself is a stressful process for all concerned. Because testing is so critical to the success of the project, it's important that the organization implements a process of celebration once it concludes to ensure that everyone gets a "pat on the back." Individuals are literally putting their jobs or even lives of their patients on the line when testing the EHR system. But careful planning, establishing good rapport with the vendor, and solid preparation of tools can ensure successful testing.

CHAPTER 8

Pre-Live
Conversion Activities

CHAPTER 8

Pre-Live Conversion Activities

In addition to system build and testing the new system, you also must address a number of pre-live data conversion activities. Pre-live conversion activities include data preparation, conversion program testing, readiness review, turnover rehearsal, implementation staffing, and actual turnover.

Organizations may carry out these activities in a variety of ways. Some will group the data preparation activities with system build and testing, and turnover rehearsal and implementation staffing with training. Others may actually not carry out some or all of these steps. A mission-critical system such as an EHR, however, deserves the most careful of pre-live conversion activities to reduce the need for dual processing and the potential for less than full adoption. This chapter

- describes steps to take to prepare data for the EHR
- ensures that conversion programs are tested in addition to the EHR system
- provides a plan for readiness review and turnover rehearsal
- identifies potential implementation staffing needs
- addresses ways to ensure life after actual go-live

Data preparation

Chapter three described the development of a conversion strategy. That discussion primarily addressed conversion for primarily historical paper-based data that would build an electronic baseline for your EHR system.

Most healthcare organizations, however, cannot start their EHR implementation with a totally clean slate of all new patients with no existing electronic data on the go-live date. Unless you are starting a brand new facility or physician practice, there will always be some current patient data in feeder systems, such as the billing systems, ancillary systems, etc. At a minimum, you must convert data for these patients into whatever format the EHR requires. More often, additional data is also prepared for use in the EHR system. A hospital will need to ensure that the EHR can access its master person index. For a physician practice, you need to prepare data in the practice management system to support the EHR. For typical hospitals and large practices, such data preparation activities may take several days or even weeks.

Figure 8.1 **Conversion strategy v. data preparation**

Conversion strategy	Data preparation
Addresses historical, paper-based data	Current data in existing electronic systems
Paper-based data may or may not be converted to electronic; generally only some portion of paper-based data are converted	All current data must be converted
Complementary processes may be used for this conversion, such as document imaging or data abstraction	Current data must be moved directly to/interfaced with new electronic system
Timing of conversion is not absolutely critical; it may be performed for some period before or for a period of time after go-live	Current data must be moved in time for go-live

© 2004, Margret\A Consulting, LLC

You may conduct data preparation in parallel with system build and testing, although typically it is performed near the end of system build or at its conclusion. This is to ensure that the data can flow smoothly through the new system. There are actually two primary steps:

1. Preparation of existing electronic data, conversion, and testing
2. Move production data from old system to new system

The first step is to prepare to convert the data and the second step is to actually conduct the conversion for the data with which the EHR system will go live.

You can convert some data in advance, such as the master person index and existing open receivables accounts. However, most healthcare organizations want to know that they will be able to continue to get lab and other diagnostic studies results, dictations, and other data during go-live, so they will have to actually move the data files over to the new system for go-live.

Conversion program testing

Just as in testing the new system to ensure that it was built properly and will process new data correctly, it is also critical to test that old data transfers properly into the EHR environment.

In some cases, a third party may be involved in this data conversion. This is very common for master person index (MPI) conversion. Often the healthcare organization will want to perform a clean up of duplicates prior to the conversion as well. In this case, it is very important for the organization to coordinate that vendor's activities with the primary EHR vendor. It is not uncommon for each vendor to have a perspective on which system is the cause of a problem that may arise. Therefore, your organization needs to be diligent about ensuring that each vendor addresses any problem thoroughly. The end result must not only be satisfactory conversion of the data, but the ability to use the data in the system.

Glitches between old and new systems are common. No matter how carefully you have performed the data preparation task or how thoroughly you tested the data conversion, there are always potential problems. Figure 8.2 provides an example of how critical it is to test all components and modules of all applications that use any data.

Figure 8.2	**Example of data conversion problem**

A new EHR system is implemented, in which data from an admission-discharge-transfer (ADT) system regarding information about patient allergies was captured and stored in preparation of it being fed to the EHR system. An interface was built between the two systems and tested. Allergy data was found to be flowing smoothly to the new system and would appear on the correct screens. However, when the data were processed against decision support rules, the data could not be read by the rule. It was determined that the decision support module used a slightly different data dictionary than the module used for data entry.

© 2004, Michael R. Cohen

Readiness review and turnover rehearsal

Because it is so important to ensure that work goes smoothly once the live system is "turned on," many organizations develop a final checklist to make sure that everything is truly ready. In essence, go-live is not just flipping a switch but carefully constructing a plan in which each function of the new system is turned on and runs in parallel with the old system. Once organizations are sure the new system is running properly, they may then turn off the old system

Readiness review

Some organizations use a highly detailed checklist at the point of pre-live. Others use the project plan and go over every detail on it. Still other organizations use a high-level checklist, such as identified below, and return the more detailed project plan steps only as necessary. Five readiness review steps include the following:

Step one: Make sure that all modules of the applications are fully built out, workflow and process redesigns complete and working, and backup and downtime procedures are in place.

You'll also want to ensure that all users received training, were assigned access privileges, and have changed their default passwords. Although you might assume that these steps were completed prior to pre-live activities, checking actual against project plan ensures that assumptions are accurate.

Step two: Verify that all human-computer interface and other peripheral devices are installed, placed in the proper location, and in working order. Check, for example, that there is sufficient paper in printers, cables are connected from workstations, handheld and portable devices secured, cabinets built or installed to hold devices, carts acquired and set up for "computer on wheels" (often referred to as COW), and wireless devices have fully charged batteries.

Step three: Make sure all modules are set to produce data validation reports, backup lists, and perform other processes needed for parallel runs. Even if the EHR is phased in per unit and the intent is not normally to produce paper backups, it is important that these be run during the go-live conversion. They serve as backup in the event you need them, and they serve to validate that the EHR is functioning properly. For example, if you implement CPOE as one of the EHR applications, you should print the orders entered into the system and validate them against those received in each department.

Step four: Ensure that existing applications are either not affected or affected only as intended by the EHR. An EHR is a clinical system, but many of the functions performed generate charges, work orders, task lists, and other pass-offs that other, existing systems must receive and process. Even though you should have tested each thoroughly during formal testing, you need to validate them during the actual go-live.

Step five: Ensure that all functions set to cease after go-live actually are ready to stop and, if so, that they ceased properly. Although you will need some parallel processing for a short time, it is not appropriate to run dual systems for very long. It is important to know when they are ready to be turned off and that they have been turned off properly.

Turnover rehearsal

Many organizations will actually rehearse go-live in the test environment. Timing of various procedures may be critical, so you must test it. Each person who has a role to play in the go-live should feel confident that he or she understands the tasks and can perform them as necessary.

Implementation staffing needs

A team of implementation specialists from the vendor or a consultant will normally assist in the many activities associated with implementation. The EHR vendor can frequently advise you on how many additional support personnel you need. This is not the time or place to skimp. Not only will inadequate staffing lead to delays and extensions, when you actually implement the EHR system, the inability to thoroughly perform the critical checks described above could be dangerous.

Go-live support

A good rule of thumb for go-live is to "expect the unexpected." Despite careful planning, checking, and rechecking, there is always something that can happen or even go wrong during actual go-live. Part of the go-live support should be a strong communication mechanism that gets support staff to attend to problems immediately. There should also be contingency plans, such as an approved workaround plan until you correct the problem, in the event that you can't fix something immediately.

For clinicians who are new to using computers, having adequate support for getting help and responding to questions reduces the inevitable stress of go-live. Even if all staff members have undergone their training, it will still be slow going for the first several days and even weeks. Much like first impressions, a bad go-live can significantly reduce user trust and will generally lead to considerable resistance.

Staffing considerations should include the following:

- Who will provide assistance to users during the first few days/weeks of go-live? Many organizations have their vendor supply trainers to provide users with side-by-side support. Some vendors have their staff wear distinctive clothing so users can easily spot them and quickly solicit them for help. The organization's super users might also want to consider doing this during the go-live period.

- How will trainers and other staff provide support on the day of go-live? This is an especially critical decision if the organization expects users to access the system in examining rooms and other patient care areas. Be sure your vendor has signed a business associate contract and that the vendor's staff members have received whatever training your healthcare organization may require for privacy and security.

- Will the organization approve overtime for staff who provide assistance, for those who are actually using the system for the first time and find it slow going initially, or to supplement staff who are using the system for the first time?

- Are both the vendor's technical support personnel and your IT staff on-call and ready for immediate response to any technical issues? Although testing and training attempts to anticipate every conceivable problem, there is a rare go-live that doesn't encounter some technical problem, even if minor.

- What have the patients been told? Some organizations literally put signs up indicating that their computer system is "under construction," so that patients will understand why some functions may take a bit longer or why there are suddenly many more people around. For a large organization, it may be appropriate to be sure that patient liaisons are fully trained and ready to respond to questions. Some patients might ask questions related to confidentiality and security. Others might ask more sophisticated questions about where and how their data are stored, how they might get access to data, or even how they can contribute to their records. Many patients are very computer savvy, using computers at work, school, or home. Adopting an EHR may be just the trigger that encourages patients to want to send e-mail to their physicians or develop a personal health record. Organizations should anticipate these questions, and have ready policies and scripts to handle them.

Patient load

Other staffing considerations include reducing patient load so that existing staff can manage the new system.

In some cases, hospitals will time their EHR implementation when they anticipate lower occupancy rates or emergency department visits. This will vary by location and type of hospital. Sometimes holidays are good times for go-live. In other locales, it might be off-season periods that are best.

In many physicians' practices, it's wise to reduce the patient load for a few days or weeks during EHR go-live so that physicians have adequate time to become accustomed to actual use.

Life after go-live

There may be the desire to breathe a sigh of relief and go back to business as usual after go-live, but you still have much to do. Chapter 10 addresses the need for celebration and lessons learned, but you must also address other more mundane tasks, such as follow-up, documentation, reconciliation of outstanding issues, debriefing, and turnover.

Follow-up

Follow-up is essential to ensure that the EHR is not only working after go-live but is adopted as intended. The EHR encompasses numerous functions and processes. During vendor selection, quality and process improvement activities, and even system build, testing, and training, much attention is devoted to these functions and processes. Once implemented, many organizations assume that the new functions and processes will be used as planned and that benefits will automatically accrue.

Unfortunately, adoption of new functions and processes does not always go as planned. You need to monitor all functions and processes to evaluate not only for accuracy but for effectiveness as well. Figure 8.3 provides an example of how such functions and processes may not always be adopted as planned.

The example in Figure 8.3 illustrates the need for regular follow-up audits. Don't waste time waiting to identify that there is a lapse in adherence to a new process or that a workaround had been created. Early identification of such issues can help identify the need for retraining or some other adjustment.

Figure 8.3	**Example of process not improved**

A new medication administration module was implemented as part of an EHR system. Nurses were given tablet computers on which to record medication administration at the bedside. On one nursing unit, the nurses continued the old process of recording medication administration on notes that they took back to the nurses' station to enter at a desktop. Because the data were entered, there was no red flag that indicated anything was wrong. However, when medication administration error rates were reviewed later, it was found that there was no improvement in the number of errors, although improvement was anticipated. Fortunately, the organization decided to conduct an audit of the situation and was able to identify that old processes had not been changed. When nurses were queried, it was identified that the tablets were heavy and there was no place to put them during the actual administration of the medication. As a result, the hospital experimented with giving nurses personal digital assistants (PDAs) that could be dropped into a pocket and with new bedside stands that had a drawer that could be pulled out and used to rest the tablet. These measures were found to be successful.

© 2004, Margret\A Consulting, LLC

Adjustments, however, may need to be in the form of continual change management. Figure 8.4 provides another example of change that was not initially accepted.

Figure 8.4	Need to manage change

A patient care documentation system was designed to use personal digital assistants (PDAs) for nursing documentation on nursing units. Although many nurses took readily to the PDAs, several nurses complained that it was difficult to see the data on the PDA. An analyst was dispatched to evaluate the situation. At first, the analyst noticed that each of these nurses wore glasses. It was suspected that the problem, perhaps, was that the font was too small or the screen was not lit properly. Tests, however, revealed that the workstations on the nursing unit actually used a smaller font than the PDA for its prompts. Nurses were shown how to adjust the backlighting on the devices. A support staff person also followed the nurses during several shifts to determine whether there were any other problems. During this time, the nurses continuously asked if they were entering data correctly. The analyst decided that there actually was nothing wrong with the device or the nurses' eyesight, but that they were older nurses who needed reassurance that they were using the system properly. It took them longer to accept the change, and they needed special attention to do so.

© 2004, Margret\A Consulting, LLC

Follow-up auditing can also reveal where new users may not have fully understood directions, where self-training was incomplete, or even where the new process was poorly designed.

Direct inspection is not the only method for follow-up auditing. A plan to have routine statistical reports can provide good information. For example, access controls and audit trails should be able to identify the device (and hence the location) from which persons are entering data. For the examples in Figures 8.3 and 8.4, audit trails could have suggested a problem if the analyst was aware that the nurses were using desktops or workstations at the nurses' station instead of the handhelds.

Documentation

Another post-go-live step should be to ensure that all documentation about the system is fully developed. This is a step many hate, but as with health care itself, documentation is critical for ongoing maintenance, planning updates, meeting contractual obligations, and providing documentary evidence of performance. There needs to be documentation of policies, procedures, instructions, rules, code changes, upgrades, patches, reinstatement of controls, and other components of hardware installation and software development.

In some cases, healthcare organizations have adopted technology to help perform documentation for change management. Enterprise change management (ECM) systems provide complete traceability of software changes, even across multiple platforms.

Reconciliation of outstanding issues

Proper documentation will also help track and identify any outstanding issues that remain after go-live in order to achieve their reconciliation. Even though the vendor will also log issues, your log reflects your comfort level with whether something has been fixed or not.

Some organizations use help desk or other similar software to help track issues and their resolution. For each issue, the software will literally create a ticket. Both the organization's project manager and its vendor can use the ticket to sign off once the issue is resolved. They also can use the ticket to communicate issues that need to be escalated within either organization.

Debriefing

Reviewing what went smoothly and what did not go smoothly during the implementation may seem like putting salt on old wounds, but it can be an effective means of learning from mistakes for future implementations. A good vendor will want to do this with the client, and potentially do it after every shift or at the end of every day during the first few days of go-live. If this is performed in a constructive environment, it can be very effective in capturing ideas that will make the next implementation easier and less stressful.

In a large organization, there may be several layers of debriefing. Typically, the vendor and client's project manager and potentially the entire EHR steering committee may conduct a general debriefing. Often, then, there may be sub-level debriefings for specific staff, sometimes daily. There very likely will also be a management/executive briefing on current status and outstanding issues at the highest level.

In some organizations, the EHR is such a big event than an online bulletin is created with frequently asked questions, status reports, tips, and other information related to the EHR implementation process.

Turnover

The end result of go-live is turnover. This often comes several weeks after actual go-live and generally is a formal acknowledgement that the healthcare organization will assume responsibility for ongoing support and maintenance of the EHR from this point forward. The healthcare organization may have to sign off on the contract and make a final payment. In some cases, EHR vendors run certain tests themselves to determine whether the client is ready for turnover. This is the mark of a good vendor—after all, a client not ready to assume responsibility for the system can have problems that lead to unhappiness. Whatever the process, be aware that this is a critical milestone. Not only is there no turning back, but there is little leverage to fix implementation problems after this point. This is not to suggest that the vendor deserts you or that there is no recourse for problems in the system. However, if you have signed off that something is working to your satisfaction but then find that you made a mistake on the sign off, you may have to pay for "service" on this problem.

Real life

For much of the implementation process, implementers are working in a test environment. Some healthcare organizations even set up "war rooms" or "EHR labs" where systems are built and tested. For some technical or support staff involved in the implementation process, the real system may never be used. For others who are part of the user community but heavily invested in the planning and system build processes, the extended period of time and intensity of implementation make the go-live seem like just another test. Still others who have not been a part of the implementation activities may never appreciate what goes on in the war room or lab.

A real life EHR implementation team probably needs a dose of reality—and should be "brought up for air" for training, celebrating, and identifying lessons learned. Likewise, a dose of the war room or lab reality for users could give them a better understanding of the complexity and level of detail implementing an EHR system is all about. A real live EHR truly touches everyone.

CHAPTER 9

Training Strategies

CHAPTER 9

Training Strategies

It's important to consider your training strategies while you plan and implement the overall project—not just at the conclusion of system build or testing.

There are many aspects of training—some of which your EHR vendor can and will help you with, others of which you will want to address outside the scope of the vendor offerings. This chapter

- distinguishes among training purposes and methodologies
- describes training modalities
- addresses human resource considerations regarding training
- provides reminders about training specifics

Training purposes and methodologies

Obviously, a new system such as an EHR will require means to train users on how to use it. Project managers may overlook, however, other forms and purposes of training that are also very important. "Training" in this context is used in the collective sense to refer to all forms of imparting knowledge and skills. Figure 9.1 lists the primary purposes of training and summarizes methodologies appropriate for each purpose.

Figure 9.1	Training purposes and methodologies

Training purpose	Applicable training methodologies
Introduction—intended to introduce the concept of EHR into the organization, generate interest, and reduce fear.	• Scripted statements for managers and supervisors to use in meetings concerning the organization's intent and policies on staff retention and recruitment • Newsletter/brochures/intranet quips about EHRs, their purpose, and organizational intent • Reading material about benefits and realities of EHRs
Education—designed to explain the features and functions of EHRs and provide a baseline of skills for new users.	• Newsletter/intranet articles about EHRs • Sources for additional information • Conference/trade show attendance by key personnel with the intent of sharing education • Product demonstrations on-site • Classroom instruction for steering committee members on features and functions, roles and responsibilities, project planning and change management
Briefings—primarily for department heads, executive leadership, board members, and potentially union representatives and the press to acquaint them with concepts, costs, and benefits; provide status reports; and describe actual results, including successes and lessons learned.	• Short presentations to specific groups • Short memos on progress • One-on-one meetings as necessary to address issues
Training—the actual instruction on how to perform tasks. These tasks would include not only how to use the EHR itself, but how to perform any and all implementation tasks.	• Basic training in operating computers through a learning center or coaching • Training courses at vendor sites or by vendors in-house • Courses on specific skill sets at vendor sites or schools • Training manuals (online and offline) • Hands-on training sessions in classrooms in test environment • Live hands-on training at the work site in production environment • Self-training on intuitive components of the system with online training/help desk support

Figure 9.1 ███████████ **Training purposes and methodologies (cont.)** ████████████

Support—reminders and skill development for continual usage.	• Coaches and trainers available during go-live • Online help • Help desk • Intranet: frequently asked questions (FAQs), tip sheets • Scripts

© 2004, Margret\A Consulting, LLC

As illustrated in Figure 9.1, there are multiple training purposes and methodologies—each suitable for different audiences and use at different times within the overall EHR project.

When planning the EHR implementation, you should always remember that training is both expensive and critical.

An organization that does not develop awareness of the EHR project early on is violating one of the key principles of change management, which may have an impact throughout the rest of the project and beyond. A lack of trust is one of the most difficult issues to overcome in any environment.

Without adequate training, those who must carry out the most sensitive and complex of EHR components can make grave errors that will take considerably more time and resources to identify and correct later.

If users are not adequately trained—in the manner most comfortable for them—they will not adopt the system as desired, often creating workarounds that do not produce benefits and may actually set the organization back.

Unfortunately, many organizations get to the point of training and find that there are cost overruns they want to make up by cutting training costs, or are tired of diverting funds to the project and may not fully support the training budget. Vendors often sell systems on the premise that they are intuitive and easy to learn—suggesting that training is not that important. But for staff that have little experience with using computers, let alone sophisticated systems such as EHRs, it is imperative that training be commensurate with the complexity of the system and the desired outcomes.

In addition to planning and sticking to an appropriate EHR training budget, there are also ways to create inexpensive yet effective training modalities.

Training modalities

Some of the most effective training modalities are those that are also the least expensive. When planning training modalities, however, remember that different people learn in different ways. It is not a good idea to rely solely on one training modality, or even on one training modality for a given purpose or group of trainees. Some lessons learned include the following:

- Executives and board members tend to like very short briefings, with a somewhat more detailed written follow up to which they can refer if desired. The short briefings give them the opportunity to be informed without going into depth, but also provide them the opportunity for asking questions that a similar-in-length document would not provide.

- Managers and supervisors like to have an orientation to what they must train on so they are comfortable that they have more information than their subordinates and can respond to questions. Some managers and supervisors do well enough with solely written materials and access to related materials and resources. Generally, these are managers that have some computer savvy or are experienced through previous employment or self-interest in EHR systems. However, it is still important to ensure that managers and supervisors convey a consistent message, hence the idea of using train-the-trainer or scripts. There may be managers that are less than enthusiastic about an EHR and might impart that message to their departments in their presentation method. Other managers may believe they understand the EHR because of past experience but actually may have bad habits or have used different or older systems.

- Individuals who are targeted to become super users will have a natural inclination to using systems and will probably do considerable research on their own, including the potential for using the system ahead of the rolled out functionality. It is important not to dampen the super users' enthusiasm, but they may require some reigning in. They also may not be as understanding or compassionate when it comes to training others. Super users are not necessarily those who received instruction through train-the-trainer, and they may well benefit from such training.

- Although there is considerable variation, there is general consensus that nurses prefer to learn in groups, often with instructors, and in relatively short takes with the ability to apply what is learned to the actual activity very soon after their training. They tend to be compassionate with others, and willing and interested in helping each other. Unfortunately, this modality is among the most costly, and because of the volume of nurses you must train, it will be very expensive. If instructor-led training sessions are too costly and time-consuming, train-the-trainer sessions can be an alternative. An even less expensive approach, if available from the user, is an interactive, online set of session where users can learn and directly apply their new skills.

- Physicians tend to be opposite nurses in their training preferences. They generally prefer one-on-one training and even online training (at least, once they have mastered the initial log on). They prefer to do the online training at home or in their own offices during "off" hours. It is not that physicians are unwilling to help others, but they have a tendency to feel inadequate if they don't know something—even if they could not be expected to know. Honor their preference for "private" learning sessions to the extent feasible or it will be difficult to engage them in adoption of the system. Once they have mastered fundamentals, they do become more willing to seek help from others, such as super users, peers, or "their nurses."

- Videos, group activities, boot camps, and other training modalities are often not applicable or used for EHR training.

Human resource considerations

As mentioned in the previous section, training can be a costly proposition. The primary training costs are generally not trainers or training materials but the need to free staff time for training. For many healthcare organizations, training means overtime or adding relief staff. IT staff will need coverage when they attend vendor training seminars, just as nurses, technician, therapists, and others will need coverage for their patient care responsibilities.

In a union environment, training must adhere to union rules. Even if there are no unions involved, it is a good idea to work with human resources experts to establish the training policies.

User training
Consider the following other human resource training issues:

- Will staff be required to gain a specified level of competency? How will the organization measure competencies?

- What happens if a staff member undergoes training but fails a test or other measure of competency? Will the organization require the person to retrain on the same materials? Will it make a coach available? Will it take other aides or measures?

- As part of celebration of success, will the organization give employees certificates of training or competency achievement? Are these transferable to other organizations?

- If training is provided and a staff member leaves, are there restrictions on future employment opportunities built into staff agreements? (This is primarily an issue for those who receive extensive training from the vendor and then leave to go to work for the vendor. This is often covered in the vendor contract for acquiring the EHR system.)

- Does training lead to a pay increase? (Generally it does not; however, it could depend on the training. Training to perform the same duties using the EHR generally should not be the basis for an increase; however, you may potentially need to compensate training to acquire new knowledge and skills to perform different duties. Some organizations create EHR administrators for various departments whose new jobs are totally devoted to EHR build, training, and ongoing maintenance. Alternatively, not accepting the training could put an employee at risk for not being redeployed.)

- How will the organization compensate affiliated physicians for their time in learning the hospital's system, if at all? Are there physician champions who may ultimately be employed to perform as medical directors of information systems or medical informaticists?

Privacy and security training and awareness

Part of EHR training will also include information on privacy and security considerations. As many potential EHR users will not have had access to information systems in the past, the organization must create many new access privileges or make modifications to existing privileges. Users need training on how to use the system and how to apply the privacy and security rules.

The EHR potentially opens a whole new world to people, but they must understand restrictions that apply to this new world. This includes confidentiality of individuals, appropriate use of the Internet, file safety, virus protection, and password creation. Users should understand that there are audit controls and that the organization will monitor their use of the system. Many organizations place warning banners on their systems to this effect. Although not necessarily the task of the EHR project team, it should ensure consistent application of sanctions associated with use and disclosure of protected health information.

Retraining

Users may periodically need retraining, if there are upgrades or new modules added. This can generally be performed in an online session. However, monitor training to ensure that it is actually performed. Hold supervisors and managers accountable for staff members who do not take applicable training. This is actually no different than any other training and retraining requirements for blood-borne pathogens, diversity, or other topics mandated for healthcare worker training.

In addition, if audits reveal that the organization is not achieving benefits or not implementing new workflows and processes, it may have to retrain users. Although online training may be available for this purpose, usually there are specific issues the organization must address for each such user. Each will need specialized training.

Training requirements

Training for the EHR is essential, no matter at what level or with what modality. Plan and properly execute training just as you do other parts of the EHR implementation.

Sequencing of training depends on what training is needed for whom. In general, however, just-in-time training is best. For IT staff, conduct training as you anticipate the need for tasks on infrastructure preparation, system build, and testing.

For EHR users, conduct training at various strategic times. Some training on EHRs in general can help users who are involved in workflow redesign and process analysis. Some training will need to precede testing for users involved in testing. In general, however, there will be a large group of people to train once the system is ready for pre-live activities.

Celebration of Success and Lessons Learned

C H A P T E R   1 0

Celebration of Success
and Lessons Learned

Throughout this book we have stressed the importance of celebrating success. Whether you reach a milestone, sign off on acceptance testing, or individuals complete training, there are many opportunities to recognize those who help make the EHR implementation successful.

The EHR is also a complex and multi-dimensional undertaking. There are always lessons learned. Because vendors will continually refine and add to the EHR system and there are many others who are not as far along, documenting your lessons learned—for yourself and to share with others—can be immensely helpful.

This chapter

- offers suggestions for meaningful celebration of EHR success
- identifies potential ways for external recognition
- describes the importance of identifying lessons and learning from them
- discusses steps in performing a benefits realization study
- helps you plan for the next upgrade, module, or application that continues your EHR success

Celebration of success

Whether implementing an EHR or not, the world is moving at an ever faster pace and few people seem to be taking the time "to smell the roses" or give someone a "pat on the back." In an EHR environment, the result of not recognizing individuals for their contributions or celebrating successful milestones may be a less than desirable adoption rate or workarounds that result in less than desirable improvements. Celebration of success is a fundamental component of change management, but it also must be sincere and performed for success—not a matter of routine. Although it seems like celebration should come naturally and therefore does not need its own chapter in an EHR book, celebration does not always come easily or is, indeed, forgotten in hectic times and places. There are several ways to accomplish celebration in a healthcare organization.

Build into project plan

Make reviews to celebrate success actual tasks on the project plan. Be cautious, however, about celebrating only for the sake of celebrating. People will recognize when celebration is genuine and when it is another task to check off on the project plan. Noting key points for conducting a review to determine whether the celebration is appropriate can be helpful as the project gets underway, as there are many activities and many people involved.

What parts of the process you should celebrate is a matter of individual organizational discretion. Certainly you could view each milestone on the project plan as a potential point for review and celebration. As organizations become more used to—and comfortable with—celebrating success, celebration will also become more spontaneous.

Vary who, what, why, where, when, how

It may seem like a good idea to plan a pizza party at the conclusion of every milestone, but any single activity can become rote. It is important to vary what is done. Some considerations include the following:

Who is celebrated and who does the celebrating
Although the project manager may have it on the project plan to review for celebration, it should not be the project manager who is solely doing the celebrating. Instead, the project manager should remind a manager or supervisor that one of the employees has performed admirably or greatly contributed to some activity relating to the EHR implementation. The project manager can communicate the milestone, but the celebration should come from the person who is most affected.

Praise from others than a manager or supervisor can also be extremely effective. Depending on what was accomplished, it may be that an executive provides a special greeting to the individual in the hallway or writes a letter of commendation. It may be appropriate for the physician champion or one of the steering committee members to acknowledge a successful or important activity.

Celebrate teams as well as individuals. This builds team spirit and cooperation. It can be beneficial to recognize cross-functional and inter-departmental teams, especially when each are responsible for an information system and didn't share information or even where there has been some animosity because interfaces don't work well.

Don't forget the vendor when you plan celebrations. Yes, you are paying for the vendor's services, but you also pay your staff. Any individual who accomplishes a task on time, or goes out of the way to do something, and turns around a problem situation should be the target of a "thank you" or more.

Hopefully the project manager will also be the recipient of some much-deserved recognition. Certainly if a culture of celebration is instilled into the organization, recognizing the project manager's efforts will also happen.

Finally, do not forget those who are not directly involved in the EHR project. Early in the project before users are trained, it may be appropriate to share some of the celebrations with the users, so they can anticipate a positive experience and look forward to recognition when they get to the point of training and adoption. However, there will still be many who will not become users, and who may actually fear for their jobs. An example might be the file clerk who is concerned that the EHR means a dismissal. Celebration for these individuals could be a bitter pill to swallow. In such cases, it may be appropriate to find ways to celebrate when they have learned new tasks or applied for new jobs within the organization. This is actually more than celebrating but planning ahead for staffing needs.

What is celebrated

What is celebrated is an important consideration. As previously noted, celebration for the sake of celebrating is not positive reinforcement. Instead, you need to consider or conduct a formal review of what you've accomplished before you provide the party planners. What is celebrated, however, does not have to be a huge milestone. It can be the accomplishment of any small task along the way that made it easier to conduct the next set of tasks, that contributed to avoidance of a problem, or that offered a unique suggestion for how to do something better. Of course big milestones will be cause for bigger, more formal celebrations.

Why recognition is afforded

In an EHR project people are usually recognized because they did something that helped advance the project. Although this is a good reason, don't overlook other reasons. Reasons that are personal—such as helping a coworker overcome a problem—or for the good of the patients—such as recognizing how an extra few seconds to perform a step can mean a difference—are outstanding reasons for recognition. The more varied the reasons for recognition, the more likely people will be responsive and want to contribute to the project.

Where recognition is afforded

Decide whether you will privately or publicly conduct the recognition. Some people may feel embarrassed if they are singled out for a contribution, yet others may feel left out if you publicly recognize another group and not them. Once again, building recognition and celebration into the culture of the organization will make it more natural. Seeing some get recognized helps others provide recognition as well. Working with the individuals and their supervisors or managers can help determine the most appropriate recognition modality.

Some organizations actually take specific steps to provide public recognition. There might be an EHR project success story of the week posted to the organization's intranet, a list of special contributors in a newsletter, or a plaque in the lobby recognizing the work of teams. Sometimes holding an event, such as a pizza party, ice cream social, or other gathering is needed just to get everyone excited about a major milestone accomplishment.

When recognition is afforded

Recognize an individual or team or celebrate a milestone as close to the achievement date as possible. Obviously, after a long night of sitting up during last minute go-live preparation is not the time for a party. But a few days or a week later at the most is appropriate.

Don't forget to make accommodations for those who must remain on duty during the event—either through providing relief so they may attend in part or hold events on a rotating basis so you can involve every shift. One hospital held a "midnight madness" party for everyone who had to stay late through the go-live.

How to celebrate

Keep in mind that a few words from the CEO—even in an ad hoc encounter—can be as powerful, and maybe even more so, as a big bash. Budget for celebrations, but they should not cost an unrealistic amount of money. Again, letters of commendation or announcing a special contribution at a meeting cost nothing. Other forms of celebration have very minimal cost. One physician's office gave every employee a baseball cap the day the contract was signed to acquire the EHR. This was a thank you for the work done in vendor selection as well as to let everyone know they were becoming a part of the implementation team.

External recognition

Organizations usually conduct celebrations or individually recognize the persons and teams that helped make the EHR happen. But the organization itself can deserve recognition. The EHR is generally considered a risky endeavor and not one that every organization undertakes. Although there is momentum growing for adoption of EHRs, there is no regulation mandating adoption. As such, the healthcare organization might choose to publicly recognize its efforts. This is good marketing and promotion. It identifies for the public that the organization is moving forward with efforts to be productive and effective. It can help recruit staff. It also gives individuals within the organization a sense of pride and ownership that they belong to an organization that not only put them through this rigorous change process but is also being recognized for its accomplishments.

Award and recognition programs

Healthcare organizations may apply to several award and recognition programs. The Healthcare Information and Management Systems Society (HIMSS) manages the Davies Award of Recognition for Exemplary Implementation of an EHR. This award requires an application and a site visit. It is an annual awards program in which the recipients must make formal presentations of their EHR implementation. The application is quite rigorous, including a section in which you must quantify value to the organization.

There is also a "Most Wired" recognition program conducted by the Health and Hospital Network (H&HN) publication. Other publications focus on specific types of recognition, and some focus on individual contributions.

Other forms of recognition

Other ways the organization can recognize its EHR success are through publication of success stories/lessons learned. Trade publications want to publish articles that will help others overcome resistance, learn about a new way to do something, or describe innovative approaches. Writing an article may seem like a lot of work, but a public relations department can help significantly. A few well-placed articles not only provides evidence that an organization is moving forward with an EHR but also provides personal recognition for those within the organization who are members of the trade group.

Seeking grant funds is another opportunity, not only for recognition but to potentially fund additional EHR efforts. Often granting organizations want to see evidence that the healthcare organization can manage the grant funds and will put them to good use. If an organization is not involved in research where grant writing is commonplace and managing grants become a matter of routine, success with a project of the scope and complexity of an EHR may be just the project that would trigger a successful grant award.

Don't forget to engage the organization's board of directors. Although you may consider the board an "internal" group, many boards have members from the community who can publicize the successful EHR in ways the organization itself cannot. At a minimum, it can solidify the importance of the EHR to positive outcomes that employers will appreciate when it comes time for negotiating healthcare service contracts.

Vendor awards are yet another potential form of recognition. A vendor that receives an award from an organization such as Towards the Electronic Patient Record (TEPR) does so only by having a successful client base. Such an award reflects well on the organizational clients. Vendors can also write case studies that provide this type of recognition (although you may want to consider this as a negotiable item that you'll address only when you are completely satisfied with the vendor's performance).

Lessons learned/course correction

Although the end goal of any EHR system is always success, part of the ongoing implementation process as well as post-implementation review is to identify problematic areas and capitalize upon them as a means to learn how to avoid such mistakes or problems in the future. It is also important to continuously review the outcomes of the EHR in the event that problems arise that need correction. Some of the award programs actually require the organization to identify lessons learned.

It is not the intent of describing lessons learned to criticize either the organization or the vendor. Instead, the purpose is to help your organization for the future and to help others avoid your mistakes or determine ways that might help them address similar ones.

Identifying and tracking lessons

One way to track lessons learned is through an issues log. This was described under project planning and then again under pre-live conversion activities. But not every issue warrants the label "lesson learned." Many issues are merely the tedious minutia that comes from smart humans implementing dumb computers. Review the issue log to determine whether there is a pattern of failures or steps individuals or teams aren't taking or need addressing as the project goes along. For example, the issues log may help you identify whether there is always a certain brand of equipment that is problematical, or a certain type of step in every process that takes longer to implement.

Debriefings are another important source of identifying lessons learned. This is typically the time when patterns of problems rise to the top or when people coming together recognize that there might have been a better way. For example, would it have been better to perform an activity during second shift instead of third, or should you have trained on the job rather than in a classroom for a certain type of procedure?

After you've implemented the system and put away your project plan and issues log, it is wise to create some other form of tracking for lessons learned. This is when hindsight is at its best, but also when people are tired of documenting every little detail. There should, in fact, be a formal process for auditing the results of an EHR implementation. This ongoing process should compare expected outcomes and benefits against actual. It should also review planned process changes against actual.

Documenting the lessons also provides for corporate history. Figure 10.1 is an example.

| Figure 10.1 | **Corporate history lesson** | |

One hospital relates how it implemented a CPOE system and turned on every single decision support rule supplied by the vendor, only to have an outcry from physicians who couldn't get their documentation performed because they spent so much time addressing the rules. Lesson learned: Implement only the rules that are truly critical.

Although you might expect that such a lesson would remain with the organization for some time to come, a new team implementing a nursing documentation system ended up doing exactly the same thing. Nurses were outraged that they had no control over how they could override elements of the reporting by exception pathways that were implemented.

© 2004, Margret\A Consulting, LLC

Learning from lessons

Identifying lessons learned not only means tracking the potential solution, but learning how to recognize a similar—but not exactly the same—issue in the future. After all, once the organization learns that turning on all the rules in a CPOE system is a bad idea, it will never do that again. Except, the hospital did something very similar when putting in place its nursing documentation system. (In addition, other organizations would benefit from learning about these lessons.)

Identify and track the underlying lesson surrounding a problem area. One lesson from the above example might be that doing "all" of anything is rarely a good idea. Being judicious and testing is generally better. Furthermore, you need to introduce anything new in phases when you implement any project or system. A clinical decision support system (CDSS) significantly impacts users. Anything that impact users is probably a target for phased implementation. Figure 10.2 illustrates another example of such a lesson learned.

| Figure 10.2 ▆▆▆▆▆▆ | **Need for teaming lesson** | ▆▆▆▆▆▆ |

An organization implementing the nursing documentation component of an EHR decided to let each nursing unit decide when it was ready for full EHR go-live. After all, it felt, who better to know when they were ready than the actual users?

In this case, a couple of units were very anxious to adopt the EHR. Unfortunately, they did so prematurely, experiencing a number of problems along the way. Once burned, the rest of the units were gun shy and no one wanted to go next.

In this case, the lesson learned was that a complex implementation is a team effort and the team with a full range of expertise should determine readiness. (Certainly the IT department should not make the go-live determination either.)

© 2004, Margret\A Consulting, LLC

Course correction

Lessons learned are primarily for the betterment of the organization. Course correction should be the result of auditing for inconsistencies or less than desirable outcomes. Clearly the hospital that turned on too many CPOE rules quickly corrected that by turning them all off and then deciding which to turn on and in what sequence. The organization that experienced the nursing unit go-live problem settled the issue by convening teams, using a checklist to ensure that everything was actually ready for go-live, and prioritizing go-live based on objective criteria.

Sometimes course correction, however, is not as straightforward as these examples suggest. One of the most insidious lessons to learn from and correct is when users start to create workarounds for new processes, or—worse—demand customization of the system to reflect current processes. Sometimes these scenarios can be difficult to identify. Some customization is desirable and necessary. Most EHR systems are built so they organizations can customize them to their needs. But there is a fine line between customizing to accomplish better outcomes and customizing to accommodate people unwilling to make change. Once again, a team approach can be helpful. Figure 10.3 provides a good example of the need for team pressure.

| Figure 10.3 ▬ | **Team pressure supports lesson** ▬ |

A hospital was in the process of implementing a new radiology information system (RIS) and picture archiving and communications system (PACS). In advance of the installation, it clearly identified workflow redesign and process changes. The goal was an integrated digital healthcare environment, with the expectation that as it replaced or added other medical devices, the new equipment would conform to the data exchange standards (from the Integrating the Healthcare Enterprise [IHE] consortium) needed to achieve interoperability between systems that process data and systems that process images.

As implementation proceeded, however, it became clear to the project manager that the effort was still viewed as a "radiology" system. Cardiology, pathology, and others that anticipated incorporating digital images of angiography, ultrasound, and other output from medical devices were left out of the workflow and process redesign issues. The result was that not only were these departments' needs not fully anticipated for future implementation, external users of the RIS/PACS were not well considered either.

Fortunately, the project manager had sufficient authority as well as responsibility and foresight to see that the organization addressed this issue. Original specifications were brought to the table and team members from other disciplines were able to cite inconsistencies between planned and actual activities. With documentation in hand, the other members of the team felt they had reasonable ground on which to make their case before it became too late and to prevent the need for course correction.

© 2004, Margret\A Consulting, LLC

A strong project manager can successfully intervene when there appears to be a potential problem brewing. However, such potential problems are not always easy to spot. In fact, they may not occur until well after implementation.

Benefits realization

One way to ensure that course correction takes place is through a formal benefits realization study. Although every organization wants to know that its EHR is achieving desired outcomes, few actually take the time and effort to do a formal study.

Some suggest that if people are happy with the EHR, there is no need to spend further effort. Figure 10.4 provides a perfect example.

Figure 10.4 ▬▬▬▬▬ **Lessons in happiness** ▬▬▬▬▬

A hospital decided to implement a document imaging system for clinician access to data. It was first used in the emergency department where there was a significant problem in gaining access to lab results that were performed a few days earlier in the hospital or outpatient department. It next planned to implement the system in the intensive care, where length of stay was affected by not having instantaneous access to results that the document imaging system could COLD feed. Finally, it was rolled out to the acute care units, where the desired benefit was improvement in charge capture where loose reports often never got into the record and therefore could not be reconciled against claims. Once implemented in each area, the system was widely hailed as a huge improvement over lost charts or loose reports that could not be found.

Although the stated goals were to reduce repetitive, and costly, diagnostic studies testing, average length of stay, and lost charges, once implemented and everyone was happy, the hospital did not go back and study whether it was achieving its original goals. However, a revenue cycle management audit 18 months later revealed that although the system resolved the lost charge problem, length of stay was the same in all areas. The organization conducted a study to determine why the new system had not met this goal. The study identified two primary factors for the problem. First, there had really been no communication associated with the goal of reducing length of stay. Second, there were no process changes that would have capitalized on the information availability. Results were available, but action was often not taken on the results any sooner than in the past.

© 2004, Margret\A Consulting, LLC

Other reasons given for not conducting a formal benefits realization study is that there are many variables that contribute to whether an EHR is successful: Is improvement due to the identification of workflow and process problems, or due to the actual changes made as a result of the EHR? Is an improvement the result of better data, more data, or the availability of better and more data? Are medication errors reduced because of a general overall awareness of patient safety issues or the actual electronic support? And, perhaps most critically, against what measures are the organizations making benefits realization studies? Are there truly comparable benchmark data available? Was time taken prior to EHR implementation to establish the necessary metrics, take measurements, and control for external factors? Figure 10.5 provides a classic example associated with benefits realization studies.

| Figure 10.5 | ███████████ | **Benefits realization study issues** | ███████████ |

A hospital instituted CPOE and electronic medication administration record (EMAR) systems with the anticipation that it would reduce medication errors. It meticulously reviewed its prior incident reports to establish benchmark data.

Simultaneously with the implementation of the CPOE and EMAR systems, the hospital also instituted an online incident reporting system and provided instructions to use the error-reporting guidelines from the National Coordinating Council for Medication Error Reporting and Prevention (NCC MERP).

Following implementation of the new systems, the hospital conducted a formal benefits realization study—only to find that medication errors increased! The key factor, of course, was that the organization instituted a new reporting system and that, in effect, the hospital had no valid benchmark data with which to compare past and current performance. This is not to suggest that the hospital should have established one project at a time—after all, if both are known to help improve quality of care, it makes sense to do both without concern for research designs. Perhaps the new guidelines were not available until after the systems had been acquired or even partially, if not fully, implemented. Indeed, part of the problem with benefits realization studies is their timeliness in a dynamic environment. However, expect that over time with both the new systems and the new error-reporting guidelines the error rate would go down—and the new systems would receive as much "credit" for success as the reporting guidelines.

© 2004, Margret\A Consulting, LLC

Planning for the future

The success of an EHR implementation is important for making future progress. Success comes in many forms, however. During implementation, success is accomplishing a task or reaching a milestone. You need to recognize individual and team efforts and celebrate accomplishments. Success is also something that organizations can and should quantify after implementation—if you take care to establish appropriate metrics and conduct accurate "before" measurements, appropriately time benefits realization studies, and account for confounding variables. If you can't accurately perform a quantitative benefits study due to too many confounding variables or too much elapsed time, then make efforts to obtain qualitative and anecdotal data on results.

Some executives say, "They've never known an information system that paid for itself," or "achieved the expected benefits." If you don't study benefits, it is impossible to determine whether there has been actual success. Planning for success needs to include planning for measuring success and celebrating it, for with such success and celebration comes the opportunity for more.